the Calendar Diet

A month-by-month guide to losing weight while living your life

BY MELINA B. JAMPOLIS, M.D.
and KAREN ANSEL R.D.
with AMI JAMPOLIS, M.S.

WAGGING TAIL PRESS, LOS ANGELES

Cover Design by Jane Teis
Interior Design by Ryan Douglass

Wagging Tail Press Los Angeles, CA

Table Of Contents

the *the* Calendar Diet

Forward

As a doctor specializing in nutrition and weight loss, I've been helping people lose weight for more than a decade. In that time, there have been many developments and lots of debate about the best way to slim down. Yet, there's one thing weight loss experts seem to agree on: for long-term success, a diet has to be livable and realistic.

It also has to show you how to manage your weight all year long. While many of us can manage a diet plan most days of the week, it can be hard to anticipate and outsmart diet roadblocks that pop up throughout the year. From 4th of July barbeques to Thanksgiving Day to Super Bowl Sunday, all year long we're bombarded with a never-ending stream of special occasions that can sabotage even the savviest dieter. Hidden in the pages of the calendar is a less obvious, but equally frustrating, challenge: monthly ups and downs in motivation that can make or break our diets. In my practice I work with my patients month-by-month to help them successfully navigate these challenges and boost their motivation – all year long.

The Calendar Diet is a year- round weight loss plan that will show you month-by-month how to drop those pounds while still living your life. In doing so, I just had one problem. I don't really cook – I'm more of a heat and eat kind of gal. I needed to find someone to develop delicious, satisfying and healthful recipes.

I love to read women's health, fitness and cooking magazines for healthy meal ideas and recipes for my patients. For the past few years, it seems like every recipe I loved was written by the same person, Karen Ansel, R.D. So I reached out to Karen and told her about this project, and she enthusiastically agreed to create all of the delicious, seasonal recipes you'll find in this book. Karen's recipes sound so delicious, they've even inspired me to whip out a few pots and pans and give them a try myself.

In addition, since I love to exercise but I'm not a certified personal trainer, I enlisted the help of my sister, Ami Jampolis, who has a master's degree in exercise science and has been whipping people into shape for years.

I know you'll find this monthly, seasonal approach to eating to be an inspiring way to lose weight and make your health a year round priority at the same time. So, let's get started and let the weight loss begin!

In good health,
Melina B. Jampolis, M.D.

one
Diet &
Monthly Guide

Introduction

The Calendar Diet's secret to weight loss is its three-pronged approach that includes easy-to-follow, seasonally inspired diet advice, healthy recipes, and exercise advice. To tie all of this together you'll find four key weight loss tools:

1. A seasonal menu plan filled with recipes made from seasonal fruits and vegetables. Not only will this give you a big nutrition boost, eating fruits and vegetables that are at their peak will help you save at the supermarket, especially if you buy locally produced items. In addition to the ingredients, the meals you'll be eating will be also tied to the season. You'll enjoy leafy green vegetables in spring, cool salads and smoothies in summer and hearty, warming stick-to-your-ribs dishes in fall and winter.

2. A month-by-month guide to tackling challenging eating situations. Every month of the year is filled with diet landmines. Super Bowl party? No problem. Our No Guilt Nachos will keep you from feeling like a middle linebacker by the end of the game. Valentine's Day? Surprise your sweetie with our quick and easy Banana & Chocolate Fondue. Summer barbeques? We'll show you how to slash calories without deprivation. And for holiday parties we'll deliver loads of tips to help you maintain your weight - or even lose weight if you really work at it.

3. Motivational tips and homework to keep you on track year round. We realize that it's almost impossible to lose weight when your motivation is low or you're faced with non-stop temptation (hello late November through December). Simply maintaining your weight during trying times is the key to long-term weight loss. Each chapter will help you identify, and work through those times of year where you're likely to be less motivated or focused.

4. A build-your-own-workout section to help you customize a fat-burning, body conditioning workout. By allowing you to mix and match exercises, you'll switch up your workout every season (or every month, if you prefer) to continually challenge yourself, improve your fitness level, and work each major muscle group in different ways to prevent weight loss plateaus. Plus, you'll also receive seasonal ideas to keep you active outside the gym year round.

What you won't find: extreme diet advice. The beauty of *The Calendar Diet* is that it's both healthful and livable. You won't cut out major food groups or battle hunger. It's a system that I personally know works based on a decade of research and experience. The plan is based on one of the healthiest, research-backed diets in the world: the Mediterranean diet, which is loaded with fresh fruit, vegetables, whole grains, fish, beans, and olive oil.

Here's a brief overview of what you'll eat:

1. Slightly more **lean protein** to control hunger, stabilize blood sugar, boost metabolism, and build and protect muscle.

2. A lot **more vegetables.** Vegetables are packed with fiber and water and low in fat so they decrease the calorie density (that translates to calories per serving) of your diet while boosting overall nutrition.

3. Mostly **whole grains** to regulate insulin levels and mobilize fat stores.

4. Moderate amounts of **healthy fat** from foods like nuts, avocado and olive to keep calories under control and boost the absorption of fat soluble vitamins like A, D, E and K.

You'll put this into action by feasting on simple, year-round meal ideas as well as 52 delicious, seasonal recipes. To make it super easy, lunch and dinner recipes are completely interchangeable. The recipes serve two, but you're encouraged to double them for healthy leftovers for lunch the next day.

Ideally *The Calendar Diet* would start in January, the biggest dieting month of the year. But if it works better for you, you can start it at any time of year. If you begin during any other month, I recommend reading the motivation tips and doing the homework exercises at the beginning of the book so that you can implement the early behavior strategies to keep you on track all year long.

If you want to see fast results and need a jumpstart, consider choosing lower carbohydrate lunch and/or dinner options or go to Appendix C for Diet Booster Tips and Plateau Busters.

Chapter One: Getting Started

Welcome to *The Calendar Diet!* Your first priority will be to start keeping a food journal. Research shows that recording what you eat every day doubles your weight loss success. Your journal doesn't need to be anything fancy – a small notebook or basic Excel spreadsheet will do the trick. Then, simply track what you eat and the time of day you ate it. If you're particularly hungry one day, or find that a certain meal is especially satisfying, make a note of it. This will help you to customize your personal weight loss plan going forward.

Many people also find that recording their mood or location helps them identify problem situations. A food journal can really help you pinpoint times or places that you may be eating more than you realize, or where you could cut back a little. I also recommend tracking your exercise too so you can make changes, if necessary, and keep tabs on your progress throughout the year.

I've found keeping a food journal really helps keep my patients on track (I use one most of the time too!) However, not everyone has time to do this, or even needs to after a while, especially if you tend to eat the same foods day after day. If this sounds like you, you can stop keeping the journal after your first month or two, so long as you're steadily losing weight. If your weight loss plateaus or you feel yourself getting off track and need to refocus, make sure to start the journal back up.

Next, flip to Appendix A, the Homework Section for your first assignment. Here you'll make a list describing what losing weight means to you, to help you set priorities and guide you through challenging eating situations. Be as specific as you can and put as much time and effort into this as possible as you'll refer back to it often throughout the next year.

Other useful tools for getting started include a food scale, measuring cups and measuring spoons. These can help refresh your knowledge of portion sizes, especially when it comes to high fat and starchy foods (see my list below). If you don't already have small plates and bowls, you may want to invest in a set. Research has proven that they are an easy way to keep portions under control and help you feel more satisfied with fewer calories.

In terms of exercise, if you belong to a gym, terrific. If not, you might want to invest in some light hand weights, exercise bands, and workout DVDs. If you're really motivated, have the space, and aren't on a tight budget, investing in a piece of home cardiovascular equipment like a bike, treadmill, or elliptical machine can help 'excuse proof' your workouts.

To design your own workout season by season, flip to the exercise section of the book where you'll find a build-your-own workout routine that includes strength training, cardiovascular exercises, and high intensity interval training (HIIT) to help you burn off those calories and lose fat.

You may also want to buy a soft tape measure to keep track of your measurements in addition to the scale. Often, the scale may not move as quickly or consistently as most of us would like, so keeping track of monthly measurements can help keep you motivated. When you get started, measure your waist, hips, upper thighs and arms, and re-measure every one to two months throughout the year. If you're just starting an exercise program, you might find that your inches drop more quickly than the numbers on the scale, which means that you're losing fat and gaining muscle, a big plus when it comes to long-term weight loss.

You might also consider investing in a home body fat scale to track changes in your body fat. Again, if you're gaining muscle and losing fat, your body fat should drop even though the numbers on the scale may not always keep pace. These changes in body composition can't be detected by the average scale, and temporary plateaus can be discouraging. If you are using a home body fat scale, it's important to weigh yourself at the same time every day to ensure that your level of hydration is roughly the same and doesn't cause your body fat and weight to fluctuate.

Finally, try to build a support network to help you stay on track year round. This can include any (or all) of the following: a health-minded friend, a doctor, a psychologist, a colleague at work who is also trying to slim down, a supportive relative or spouse, a personal trainer, a neighbor looking for a walking partner, or even an online community of like-minded people you feel comfortable sharing your ups and downs with. The more people you have supporting you, the better your chances of success!

How The Calendar Diet Works:

In my decade of helping patients lose weight, I have come to realize that the simpler I make the principles of losing weight, the better. My patients don't seem to care as much about the science – they just want to know what to eat. So to make it super easy, I've boiled the science of what to eat down to six basic principles. I've also included loads of recipes to show you how to do it deliciously.

The Six Calendar Diet Principles:

1. Eat some protein at most meals and snacks. This can include lean protein, plant-based protein (nuts, legumes, beans), or low fat or fat free dairy protein. This will help keep your blood sugar stable and control hunger throughout the day.

2. Work in water-rich foods like vegetables, non-cream based soups and moderate amounts of fruit and low fat or fat free dairy whenever possible to pump up the volume of food you consume without increasing calories. This will help you feel more satisfied both mentally and physically. Keep a close eye on added fat and high fat foods. Very small servings of these can boost calories – a lot. On the flip side, high fiber foods help you feel more full by increasing the volume of food on your plate without adding lots of calories.

3. Keep carbohydrates moderate. Carbohydrates come mainly from fruits, grains and starchy vegetables. Ideally, most of your grains should be whole grains. If you like, you can make trade-offs at each meal. If you eat more fruit (for example during the summer when fresh fruit is abundant), eat less starch or fewer starchy vegetables. If you eat more starchy vegetables (common during the fall and winter), eat less fruit and fewer grains. I recommend eating one to two fruits a day during the fall/winter and two to three fruits per day during the spring/summer months.

4. Eat 3 meals + 1 to 2 snacks per day. Breakfast should be approximately 300 calories, lunch and dinner approximately 400 calories, and snacks & desserts should be 100 to 200 calories. If you are smaller, less active, or have less weight to lose, opt for lower calorie snacks. If you are larger, younger, or more active, you may want to opt for snacks at the higher end of the calorie range.

If you're a dessert lover, no problem. I've provided a list of 100 calorie desserts to satisfy your sweet tooth. You can substitute dessert for one of your snacks, cut back on your dinner portion slightly, or choose one of the lower calorie dinner options.

You can also adjust your overall caloric intake slightly by adjusting meal suggestions. For example, if four ounces of protein are recommended but you are a larger man with more weight to lose, you can go up to six ounces of protein. I recommend not increasing starch from foods like bread, rice, pasta, and potatoes, as this can slow down weight loss.

5. Limit alcohol to 3 drinks per week (or less). If you drink more than that, you'll need to cut back on either starch, fruit or fat, which may cause you to miss out on important nutrients you'll need to feel your best. Whenever possible, skip the sugary cocktails and stick with beer, wine or alcohol with no or low sugar mixers.

6. Eat what's in season as often as possible. Each chapter will provide you with a list of seasonal fruits and vegetables as well as recipes incorporating seasonal produce. Try to experiment with a new fruit or vegetable every week (or a new way of preparing a seasonal fruit or vegetable). This will not only ensure you eat a variety of nutrient rich produce, it will also keep you from getting bored with your diet. As you read on, you'll find lots of seasonal recipes and meal ideas but you can also feel free to build your own using the foods from all of the major groups shown in the section below.

Major Food Groups and Serving Sizes

Starch & Grains

Examples: Rice, pasta, crackers, bread, potato, peas, corn, beans, oatmeal

Serving Size: ½ cup or 1 slice or 80-100 calories or 15 grams of carbohydrates

Tips:
- Make most of your grains whole grains
- Limit starch to 2 per meal and 1 per snack
- Stick to 3 starches per day to lose weight quickly

Protein

Examples: Fish, lean beef, chicken, legumes, beans, eggs

Serving Size: 1 ounce = 7 grams, 1 egg, 1/3 cup beans or legumes (also count as a starch)

Tips:
- Choose lean protein most of the time
- Remove the skin from poultry and choose the leanest cuts of meats possible
- Limit eggs to 7 per week

Fat

Examples: Oils, nuts, seed, avocado

Serving Size: 1 serving = 5 grams, 1 tsp. oi oil, 2 tsp. of nut butter, 1/8 cup nuts, 1 tbsp. seeds

Tips:
- Watch serving sizes of fat & measure oil
- Limit saturated and trans fat

Vegetables

Examples: All non-starchy vegetables
Serving Size: 1/2 cup cooked, 1 cup raw or leafy greens
Tips:
- Go for variety: especially orange and deep green

Fruit

Examples: Fresh, frozen and dried fruit
Serving Size: 1 small piece, 1/2 cup fresh or frozen, 6 oz. fruit juice, 1/4 cup dried fruit
Tips:
- Limit juice to 1 serving daily
- Watch serving sizes of dried fruit

Dairy

Examples: Milk, yogurt, cheese
Serving Size: 1 cup low fat or fat free, 1 oz. of cheese (this also counts as a fat)
Tips:
- Choose low fat or fat free milk and yogurt
- Limit added sugar in yogurt to 17 grams
- Watch portions of cheese closely

Meal Ideas

If you don't always have time (or don't feel like) cooking that's completely okay. Here are some easy suggestions and simple meal ideas that you can eat year-round without breaking a sweat in the kitchen.

Breakfast:

Aim for a combo of protein, fiber and healthy fat to fill you up and help
keep blood sugar on track all day.

Option 1: Basic Yogurt Parfait
1 cup of plain or vanilla non-fat Greek yogurt
+ ½ cup high fiber cereal (3-5 grams of fiber per serving)
+ ½ cup fresh fruit OR ¼ cup dried fruit
+ 1 tbsp. chopped nuts or seeds

Option 2: Power Oatmeal
1 cup oatmeal (cooked)
+ 1 tbsp chopped nuts or seeds
+ 2 tbsp. protein powder (add to oatmeal after cooking; mix with a little water before adding) OR ½ cup of low fat or fat free cottage cheese (on the side) OR 1 egg (on the side) OR prepare oatmeal with fat free milk

Option 3: Eggs & Toast (this is an easy option if you eat breakfast out)
1 egg + 2 egg whites
+ 1 slice whole grain toast
+ 1 tsp. butter (you can make this into a sandwich by serving on a whole grain English muffin instead, skipping the butter, and topping it off with a slice of low fat cheese or ¼ sliced

avocado. It also works as a breakfast burrito by serving it in a large low carb whole wheat tortilla)
+1/2 cup of fruit

Option 4: Super Smoothie
Combine 8 ounces of fat free milk, almond milk or unsweetened soy milk
+ 2 tbsp. of protein powder (I prefer whey protein as it may help with weight loss, but if you are a vegetarian soy protein is fine too; no sugar added; serving size should contain 12-14 grams of protein)
+ ½ cup fresh or frozen fruit
+ 1 serving of healthy fat (1 heaping tbsp. ground flaxseed OR 1 tbsp. chia seed or 2 tsp. nut butter)
+ sweetener if needed and ice to taste.

Here are some seasonal ideas for you to consider.

Winter Smoothie – Double Chocolate Peanut Butter
For those of you who love smoothies year-round
1 cup chocolate almond milk
+2 tbsp. chocolate flavored protein powder
+1 tbsp. peanut butter
+1 tbsp. psyllium husk (optional – boosts fiber content)
+ ice (no sweetener required)

Nutrition Stats: 272 cals, 7 g fiber, 19 g pro

Spring Smoothie– Strawberry Banana Chia
1 cup unsweetened vanilla almond milk
+ ½ cup plain nonfat Greek yogurt
+ 1 cup fresh strawberries + ½ small banana
+ 1 tbsp. chia seeds
+ ice & 1 tsp. sugar if needed

Nutrition Stats: 260 cals, 10.5 g fiber, 15 g pro

Summer Smoothie – Raspberry Peach

1 cup non-fat plain Greek yogurt

+¾ cup frozen peaches, roughly diced

+¾ cup frozen raspberries (or use fresh & add ice)

+½ cup orange juice

+1 teaspoon agave nectar

Nutrition stats: 272 cals, 5 g fiber, 22g protein

Fall Smoothie – Cinnamon Apple Flax

1 cup unsweetened vanilla almond milk

+ 6 ounces plain nonfat Greek yogurt

+ ½ cup unsweetened apple sauce

+ 1 tbsp. ground flaxseed

+ ½ tsp. cinnamon

+ 1 tsp. sugar

+ ice to desired thickness

Nutrition Stats: 256 cals, 4.5 g fiber, 19 g protein

On the go options

1.   High fiber cereal bar or small high fiber muffin + 1 cup non-fat Greek yogurt or a hard boiled egg + piece of fruit.

2.   A protein bar + a small non-fat latte

Lunch:

Start your meal with a non-cream based vegetable soup (see 5 minute vegetable starter soup below), salad, vegetables or even an apple whenever possible to cut calories effortlessly. You'll find plenty of seasonal recipes in the next section. If you usually eat out, be sure to check out the dining out ideas in the appendix section.

5 minute vegetable starter soup:
+ 1 can of condensed tomato soup – heated
+ 1 cup of microwaved frozen mixed veggies
+ pinch of oregano
For a more complete meal add ½ cup garbanzo beans and top with a tablespoon of grated Parmesan for a quick and easy minestrone.

Option 1: 'Lite' Sandwich
Use sandwich thins (100 calories), ½ whole wheat pita or a large low carb whole wheat tortilla. Or, if you're eating out, simply take off the top slice of bread. Load your sandwich with 2-3 ounces of lean protein like turkey, sliced chicken, lean roast beef, or tuna with light mayo. Add all the vegetables you can (romaine lettuce, tomatoes, spinach) and top with 1 slice of low fat cheese or 2 tbsp. of hummus or ¼ avocado. Serve with 1 piece of fruit, a side salad, a yogurt or a small bag of baby carrots.

Option 2: Entrée Salad
The seasonal recipe section of the book is packed with delicious salad recipes. If you'd also like to create your own, make sure it includes 3 ounces of lean protein, at least 2 cups of lettuce (anything but iceberg – romaine, spinach, butter lettuce), plenty of colorful vegetables, 1/3 – 1/2 cup of beans, and a serving of healthy fat like 1-2 tbsp. nuts or seeds or ¼ avocado or 1 tbsp. olive oil (and vinegar) to help keep you satisfied. If you don't use olive oil and vinegar for dressing, keep the dressing on the side and dip your fork in it before every bite. If you're not a fan of beans, you can have a small whole grain roll or 3 whole grain crackers on the side.

Here is my favorite quick and easy salad no cook salad:
+ 3 ounces of canned or pre-cooked sliced chicken
+ ½ cup of black beans
+ 2 tbsp. of guacamole
+ ½ cup salsa (mango salsa is a delicious summer option)
+Serve on 1 head chopped romaine lettuce

Option 3: Entrée Soup
Soup can be a savory fall and winter lunch option. Make sure yours contains lean protein like chicken or plant based protein like beans to keep you full a few hours. Top choices include minestrone, chicken and barley soup, lentil soup, and vegetarian or turkey chili. Serving sizes will vary but should equal about 250 to 300 calories. Serve with a piece of fruit or a non-fat yogurt for a satisfying and healthful meal.

If you're like most Americans' you eat nearly 30 percent of your meals away from home. If you have to eat out, or don't feel like cooking, flip to appendices B and F for tips on eating out as well as choosing frozen meals.

Dinner:

As with lunch, start off your meal with a non-cream based vegetable soup, salad, or vegetables and low fat dip or hummus (no more than ¼ cup). If you prefer, you can include slightly more protein and cut back on starchy carbs at night. If you saved room for dessert by choosing lower calorie snacks during the day, by choosing a lower calorie dinner option, or by cutting your dinner portion by 25 percent, choose from one of the desserts below. I strongly suggest limiting alcohol if you choose to have dessert. For delicious seasonal recipes, go to the next section.

Option 1: Basic Grilled Protein + Vegetables
Grill, bake of broil 4 to 6 ounces of lean protein including chicken without the skin, fish, shrimp (fresh or frozen), turkey, or lean red meat (no more than twice per week). Use spices for flavor. Serve with 1 to 2 cups of steamed (or microwaved) vegetables topped with 2 tbsp. of fresh Parmesan or sauté vegetables in 2 tsp. olive oil and garlic. Optional: Serve with ½-1 cup of brown rice, whole grain pasta, or barley.   You can also make this dish as a stir fry using 2 teaspoons canola oil and low sodium soy sauce or make fajitas (sauté green, red, yellow peppers and onions) and serve in 2 small low carb tortillas or 2 corn tortillas and top with 1 to 2 tbsp. of guacamole.

Option 2: Super Spaghetti & Meatballs
Make a healthier version of this suppertime staple by tossing together 1 cup each whole grain pasta and vegetables. Top with ¼ to ½ cup marinara sauce and 3 ounces of turkey meatballs (make sure to use lean ground turkey if you are making meatballs from scratch or buy frozen meatballs with less than 5 grams of fat per serving) and 2 tbsp. grated Parmesan.

Option 3: Entrée salad (see above)

Option 4: Entrée soup (see above)

Snack Ideas (Choose seasonal fruits when you can)

100 CALORIE (OR LESS) SNACKS

- 1 piece string cheese
- 2 large whole grain crackers + 1 triangle light spreadable cheese
- 1 cup plain or vanilla low fat or fat free yogurt (Greek is the most filling)
- 1 cup of vegetable soup
- 100 calorie pack of nuts
- Mini protein bar or ½ regular protein bar (see bar criteria below)
- ½ cup low fat cottage cheese
- 100 calorie pack of microwave popcorn
- 2 celery sticks + 1 tbsp of peanut butter or ¼ cup hummus

150 CALORIE SNACKS

- 1 piece string cheese + 1 serving of seasonal fruit
- Mini yogurt parfait: ½ cup yogurt + 1 tbsp. chopped nuts + ½ cup fresh seasonal fruit or 2 tbsp. dried fruit
- Mini seasonal smoothie: cut seasonal smoothie recipes in ½
- ½ cup low fat cottage cheese + 1 serving of seasonal fresh fruit
- 1 small apple + 1 tbsp. of peanut butter
- ½ whole wheat pita + 2 ounces of turkey + Dijon mustard + 1 leaf romaine lettuce
- 14 baby carrots + ¼ cup hummus
- 3 whole grain crackers + 1 slice reduced fat cheese
- Dr. Melina protein bar

200 CALORIE SNACKS

- Open faced tuna melt. ½ English muffin + ½ can water packed tuna + 1 slice reduced fat cheese
- 1 cup non-fat plain or vanilla yogurt + 1 tbsp. nuts + 2 tbsp. dried fruit
- Protein bar (look for at least 10 grams of protein and 3 grams of fiber)
- 1 cup of turkey chili
- Slightly larger portions of any of the 100 or 150 calorie snacks

DESSERT OPTIONS: (100 calories or less)

- 1 ounce of dark chocolate (60% cacao or greater)
- ½ cup fresh seasonal fruit plain or topped with 1 to 2 tbsp. lite whipped topping or 2 tbsp. non-fat vanilla yogurt
- ½ cup non-fat vanilla yogurt topped with 1 crumbled graham cracker square
- Frozen treat: No sugar added fruit bar or fugdsicle
- ½ sliced apple dipped in ¼ cup plain non-fat Greek yogurt + ½ tsp. cinnamon + ½ to 1 tsp. sugar OR 1 tbsp. honey
- Mini S'more – 1 graham cracker square + 1 marshmallow + 1 square of chocolate (heat in microwave or toaster oven until warm)
- Any of the 100 calorie snacks

Chapter Two: Late Winter

Technically, the winter months are December, January and February. But, seriously, who wants to start a diet in December? On the other hand, slimming down is a high priority for most of us in January. Keeping this in mind, the general game plan for The Calendar Diet is to begin in January, but feel free to start whenever it's most convenient for you.

January And February

Overview: Even though it's freezing outside your motivation is probably high after a month of indulging. No wonder losing weight is most people's number one New Year's resolution. To achieve this it's super important to stick closely to the eating and exercise program during this time to capitalize on your motivation. Research shows that having greater success at the beginning of a program often leads to the most success long term.

Now is the time to focus on keeping calories under control. Fill up on soup before meals (or have a hearty soup as your meal) and limit starchy carbohydrates. Since fewer fruits are in season now, choose root vegetables like sweet potatoes, turnips, parsnips and minimally processed white potatoes (no fries please) to get your nutrients instead.

Even though it seems like the holidays just ended, your first major eating challenge of the New Year is actually right around the corner: Super Bowl Sunday. Below is a complete strategy for navigating this daylong pizza and chicken wing fest.

During the second half of February, you may find your motivation starts to wane as the excitement of your New Year's resolution begins to fade.. You're also about to face one of the biggest chocolate challenges of the year, Valentine's Day.

If you find your focus slipping, go back to the list you created in the first part of the book to remind yourself why you're trying to lose weight in the first place. Next, set three mini goals that you would like to accomplish over the next month. They can be weight goals, fitness goals (I'm going to do 10 pushups, I'm going to increase cardio by 15 minutes three times a week), clothing size goals, consistency goals, cooking goals (I'm going to try a new recipe every week this month), anything you like. Jot them down here and check them off when you accomplish them.

1. —————————————————————————— ☐

2. —————————————————————————— ☐

3. —————————————————————————— ☐

Exercise: Flip to the exercise section to design your winter program. Since motivation is at its highest in January, try to sneak in some extra cardio if you can. You can do this at the gym, outside if the weather permits, or through a cardio DVD or home exercise equipment.

Lifestyle activity: If you're like most of us, wintertime means you'll be spending most of your time indoors. Try to focus on moving more inside whenever you can. Take the stairs, not just at work, but also at the mall, airport or anywhere else you can. You can also pump up your activity by standing while talking on the phone, walking around the mall on weekends or even bowling instead of seeing a movie. Also consider taking up a winter sport for fun on the weekends like ice skating, skiing, snow boarding.

Behavior Tip: Since your motivation is at its peak in January and the first half of February, your chances of success are high now. However, you won't be as successful if you don't have a plan. Take some time to sit down every Sunday and map out your week – go grocery shopping, plan your meals (at home and out of the house), schedule workout times in your calendar, and cook or bake meals that you can heat and eat easily on hectic weeknights. The more you plan, the greater your odds of success. While this applies all year, it's especially important to plan now to build and reinforce the habits you'll need to guarantee success for the rest of the year.

Seasonal Produce

JANUARY
Fruits:
Avocado, Grapefruit, Guavas, Kiwi, Kumquats, Lemons, Limes, Mandarins, Oranges, Pears, Tangerines.

Vegetables:
Beans, Beets, Bok Choy, Broccoli, Brussels Sprouts, Cabbage, Carrots, Cauliflower, Chard, Collards, Fennel, Garlic, Gourds, Kale, Leeks, Lettuces, Mushrooms, Onions, Parsnips, Potatoes, Radish, Spinach, Turnips.

FEBRUARY:
Fruits:
Avocados, Grapefruit, Guavas, Kiwi, Kumquats, Lemons, Limes, Mandarins, Oranges, Pears, Tangerines.

Vegetables:
Asparagus, Beans, Beets, Bok Choy, Broccoli, Brussels Sprouts, Cabbage, Carrots, Cauliflower, Chard, Collards, Endive, Fennel, Garlic, Gourds, Kale, Leeks, Lettuce, Mushrooms, Onions, Parsnip, Potatoes, Radish, Spinach, Turnips.

Holidays

Martin Luther King Day: If you have the day off, use this day as a power workout day. Plan two workouts or schedule a super active day with friends or family.

Super Bowl Sunday: We eat more on Super Bowl Sunday than any other day of the year except for Thanksgiving! Try these tips to tackle this challenging eating day:

1.   Limit starch at breakfast and lunch. You'll get plenty later on in the day. Start with a big veggie omelet instead.
2.   Plan a more intense workout early in the day before the big game begins.
3.   If you're hosting a party, great! You're in control of the menu. Make sure to have a few healthier dishes on hand to nibble on like vegetables and hummus or our No Guilt Nachos. If you're going to someone else's house, offer to bring a dish so you have something to healthy to nosh on. That makes it easier to simply have a taste of all the high fat junk food rather than filling your plate with it.
4.   If you're drinking, make sure to drink one glass of water in between every alcoholic beverage.
5.   30 minutes before the party or game, eat a protein and fiber-rich snack and drink a big glass of water to take the edge off hunger.
6. If you're really motivated to keep the damage to a minimum, eat a full meal beforehand and suck on hard candies or mints and drink calorie free beverages during the event. This isn't easy but when it comes to a big calorie fest like the Super Bowl, some people find it's easier not to get started at all.

Valentines Day:

If your sweetheart is taking you out for a special dinner, go with a lower carb breakfast and/or lunch. Then, skip the breadbasket at dinner and say no thanks to the heavy starch entrees like pasta so you can save room for dessert and/or a glass of wine. It's completely okay to politely ask your valentine to skip the chocolates this year.

If chocolates are everywhere in office, limit yourself to one and keep mints on hand to keep your mouth occupied. Since research shows that out of sight is out of mind when it comes to office treats, keep the chocolates as far away from your desk or office as possible. If you don't see it you'll be a lot less likely to eat it!

If you're making dessert for your sweetheart, try our simple Chocolate Fondue. By pairing fruit with chocolate, you get all the decadence – and volume - of a real dessert for a fraction of the calories.

Chapter Three: Spring

March

Overview: If you're just starting this diet, read the overview and behavior tips in the previous chapter. If you began your diet in January, your motivation may lag a little this month. That's totally normal! For many of us it's still cold out there, so you may find yourself indoors more often and less motivated to be active.

Your weight loss may also slow down a bit, especially since you don't have summer clothing and swimsuits on your mind to motivate you yet! Good news on the diet front: other than St. Patrick's Day, which isn't generally a big eating day, there shouldn't be too many eating challenges this month. If you're traveling with your family on spring break you may need a little strategy, so read on.

The main challenge this month is going to be staying focused on your goal and accepting the fact your weight loss may be a bit slower unless you have a considerable amount of weight to lose, are just starting your diet, or are exercising intensely and dieting strictly.

Exercise: If you've been doing your build-your-own workouts faithfully during January and February, you may want to switch things up this month and put together a new routine to keep your body challenged.

The more you do a certain type of exercise, the more efficient your body becomes at performing that exercise. That means you burn fewer calories, which can lead to weight loss plateaus. By changing things up every eight to 12 weeks, you can prevent this from happening.

So try something different – a new machine at the gym, exercising at a different intensity on the same machine, doing different weight lifting exercises, or taking a different class than you normally do once a week.

Behavior: To keep yourself motivated, go to the homework section of this book in appendix A and list five things that you accomplished over the past two months that you are proud of. Next, list at least three things that you'd like to accomplish over the next month (Example: make dinner at home three nights a week, prep food every Sunday for the month, squeeze in an hour of cardio on both weekend days). Check off each accomplishment as you reach it.

Seasonal produce

Fruits:
Avocados, Grapefruit, Guavas, Kiwi, Kumquats, Lemons, Limes, Mandarins, Oranges, Strawberries, Tangerines.

Vegetables:
Artichokes, Arugula, Asparagus, Beans, Beets, Bok Choy, Broccoli, Cabbage, Carrots, Cauliflower, Chard, Collards, Endive, Fennel, Garlic, Gourds, Kale, Leeks, Lettuces, Mushrooms, Onions, Parsnips, Potatoes, Radish, Spinach, Turnips

Holidays

St. Patricks Day – Limit the beer
Spring Break – Fast forward to the summer travel section

April & May

Overview: It's starting to warm up and you may find yourself thinking more and more about skin-baring summer clothes and swimsuits. So it's time to really focus on the diet again if you've slipped up a bit. One strategy: Consider filling up on salads before meals and also as satisfying entrees. Another is to up your cardio to kick your weight loss back into full gear and take advantage of your newfound motivation.

The only holiday you'll face in April is Easter and we have terrific breakfast recipes throughout the book for a delicious and healthy Easter brunch. If you celebrate Cinco de Mayo in May, our Shrimp Fajitas and Chicken Corn Cheddar Quesadillas will be perfect. Strawberry Stuffed French Toast is the perfect decadent, yet lo-cal treat for mom on mother's day and Pasta with Spring Vegetables or Thai Peanut Noodles will be a healthy way to enjoy a Memorial Day potluck.

Exercise: Start adding in outdoor workouts (this can be walking, or if you exercise more intensely, jogging or cycling). Make sure to challenge yourself as much as you can by making your cardio as intense as possible. If you are walking, try to find a path that has an incline. Or consider a walk/jog combo if you've never run before or have an injury that makes a long jog impossible.

Behavior: If you're extra motivated, congratulations! Planning ahead will help guarantee your success. If you're not as inspired as you'd like right now, you have two choices:

1. Focus on maintaining your weight. That way you can preserve your hard earned weight loss without having to start from scratch once your motivation kicks in again in summer.

2. Create a vision board that serves as a reminder of some (or all) of your reasons for losing weight. This can be as simple as an old photo in which you looked fit and happy, or more elaborate to include places you want to visit, things you want to buy, or even a cut out of the number that you want to see on the scale. Put the board in a place, either public or private, where you'll see it - often - so that it's a constant reminder of the direction you are headed in.

Seasonal produce

APRIL
Fruits:
Avocados, Grapefruit, Guavas, Kumquats, Lemons, Limes, Oranges, Strawberries, Tangerines.

Vegetables:
Artichokes, Arugula, Asparagus, Beans, Beets, Bok Choy, Broccoli, Cabbage, Carrots, Cauliflower, Celery, Chard, Collards, Endive, Fennel, Garlic, Kale, Kohlrabi, Leeks, Lettuces, Mushrooms, Onions, Parsnips, Peas, Potatoes, Radish, Rhubarb, Spinach, Turnips.

MAY
Fruits:
Apricots, Avocados, Blackberries, Blueberries, Boysenberries, Cherries, Lemons, Nectarines, Oranges, Plums, Raspberries, Strawberries.

Vegetables:
Artichokes, Arugula, Asparagus, Beans, Beets, Bok Choy, Broccoli,

Cabbage, Carrots, Cauliflower, Celery, Chard, Endive, Fennel, Garlic, Kale, Kohlrabi, Leeks, Lettuces, Mushrooms, Onions, Peas, Radish, Rhubarb, Shallots, Spinach, Squash.

Holidays

Easter Sunday – If you celebrate Easter Sunday, chances are you'll be having a big brunch. If you are cooking, consider one (or two) of our spring breakfast options. If not, make sure to have a little protein in the morning before heading out the door (half cup of Greek yogurt or cottage cheese is perfect). At brunch watch out for diet traps that are loaded with cheese or syrup or breakfast breads and baked goodies that are oozing with fat and sugar.

Cinco de Mayo – Mexican food can – but doesn't have to be – a challenge. Priority number one: skip the chips. Unless you have incredible willpower, it's really hard to limit yourself to just a few. Then, watch the dishes drowning in cheese or topped with creamy sauces. If you'll be eating burritos or Mexican entrees, consider skipping the rice entirely and just having beans (their smart combo of protein and fiber will keep you full for hours). Finally, limit yourself to one (or two, max) margaritas. The average margarita clocks in at around 300 calories, most of which is sugar. Better yet, try making your own low-cal version with a diet margarita mix or tequila, fresh lime, club soda and a pinch or two of sugar.

Mother's Day – If you're a mom and your family is treating you to breakfast in bed or a dinner out, why not suggest that they make one of our healthy spring recipes. Going out? Drop a few hints about restaurants you'd like to go to, mentioning the ones you know aren't going to sink your diet.

Memorial Day – Chances are there's a potluck or barbeque on your calendar sometime this weekend. For barbeque ideas, check out the summer barbeque section in the next chapter. If you're going to a potluck the most important thing you can do is to scan the entire buffet before filling up your plate. This allows you to 'budget' your calories more effectively by deciding ahead of time which foods you're going to fill up on (salad, lean protein), which foods you're going to skip, and which foods you're going to splurge a little on. One of the best things about a potluck is you actually have a say in what goes on the table, so don't forget to bring something healthy and delicious to share.

Chapter Four: Summer

June

Overview: As the weather heats up so does your motivation. After all, it's a lot easier to stay focused when you want to fit into that sundress, swim suit or shorts. To take advantage of your newfound resolve - and the lack diet buster holidays - it's time to really buckle down, before the busy summer travel and barbeque season kicks into full swing next month.

Colorful, phytonutrient packed berries are in peak season this month. Not only are they an easy way to satisfy your sweet tooth, they're also packed with filling fiber. Sneak them into meals and snacks whenever you can. Right now, you might also want to consider chooser lower carb meals or cutting back a bit on starchy carbohydrates like bread, pasta and rice to speed up your weight loss.

Exercise: Since you're extra motivated right now, why not try something new that will really challenge you? That might mean a new exercise class, a new sport, a few jumpstart sessions with a personal trainer, or finding a new and challenging hike to catapult you to that next fitness level. Now is also the perfect time to build your summer workout routine from the exercise chapter of this book (spoiler alert: your motivation will probably drop a little next month). Having a few weeks of your new workout under your belt may help keep you on track.

Behavior: If you're still feeling really inspired, you may want to start keeping a journal again to stay super focused. Go to the Homework section of the book and each week, take some time to list what weight loss has meant to you so far this year. Looking back on this list in July and August, when your motivation starts to drop, could help prevent you from falling off track.

Seasonal produce:

JUNE
Fruits:
Apricots, Avocados, Blackberries, Blueberries, Boysenberries, Cherries, Figs, Lemons, Melons, Nectarines, Oranges, Peaches, Plums, Raspberries.

Vegetables:
Artichokes, Arugula, Asparagus, Beans, Beets, Bok Choy, Broccoli, Cabbage, Carrots, Cauliflower, Celery, Chard, Collards, Corn, Cucumbers, Endive, Fennel, Garlic, Kale, Kohlrabi, Leeks, Lettuces, Mushrooms, Okra, Onions, Peas, Bell Peppers, Chili Peppers, Potatoes, Radish, Rhubarb, Shallots, Spinach, Squash, Tomatoes.

Holidays:

Father's Day - Happy Father's Day to all the dads reading this book! If you'll be having (or going to) a barbeque today, fast forward to our 4th of July strategies so you can celebrate without undoing all your hard work.

July & August

Overview: Summer is officially here. That means road trips, family vacations, and a lot less structure. In this chapter, we'll tackle travel head on and give you practical ideas for before, during and after your trip. We'll also deliver ways to trim calories at weekend barbeques, especially if you're the one doing the cooking.

The good news is that there's lots of fresh fruit in season – an easy way to effortlessly lighten up meals. When watching your weight you can, however, have too much of a good thing. If you eat a bit more fruit over the next two months, be sure not to overdo it, keeping an eye on serving sizes. Even though it's great for you fruit still has calories and the sugar in fruit, if over-consumed, can sideline your weight loss, especially if you're a woman.

Realistically, your weight loss is probably going to slow down over the next two months. So it is okay to lower your expectations - a little - especially if you're travelling extensively.

Exercise: Traveling can make it hard to stick with your exercise routine. Do your best to sneak in a workout whenever and wherever you can, even if it's just a short one. Plan active family time and squeeze in a power walk as often as possible. If you're travelling, consider throwing an exercise band in your suitcase so you can do a few resistance exercises wherever you are. Now is also a great time to think about taking up a new outdoor activity or sport that you've always wanted to try – even if it's just a weekend tennis clinic.

Behavior: Since you may be less focused than usual, it's critical to get on the scale every week for the next two months - no exceptions, no excuses! I can't tell you how many times my patients have avoided the scale when their motivation is low, only to find out that the slight tug at their waist is actually a 10 pound weight gain. Don't let this happen to you. It's okay to gain a pound or two on vacation. But if you gain more than that, try to get back on track right away, to avoid erasing your hard work and slipping further and further away from your goal.

Go back to your original list of reasons for losing weight and highlight the most important reason. If necessary, start keeping a food journal again to help you get things back under control and to keep you accountable. And don't be afraid to re-enlist the help of your support group (or expand or change it around if you current group isn't giving you the support you need).

Seasonal Produce:

JULY
Fruits:
Apricots, Avocados, Blackberries, Blueberries, Cherries, Figs, Grapes, Lemons, Melons, Mulberries, Nectarines, Oranges, Peaches, Plums, Raspberries, Strawberries.

Vegetables:
Arugula, Beans, Beets, Broccoli, Cabbage, Carrots, Celery, Chard, Collards, Corn, Cucumbers, Endive, Eggplant, Fennel, Garlic, Kale, Kohlrabi, Leeks, Lettuces, Mushrooms, Okra, Onions, Peas, Bell Peppers, Chili Peppers, Potatoes, Radish, Rhubarb, Shallots, Spinach, Squash, Tomatoes.

AUGUST
Fruits:
Apples, Avocados, Blackberries, Figs, Grapes, Lemons, Melons, Nectarines, Oranges, Peaches, Pears, Plums, Pomegranate, Raspberries, Strawberries.

Vegetables:
Arugula, Beans, Beets, Broccoli, Cabbage, Carrots, Celery, Chard,

Collards, Corn, Cucumbers, Endive, Eggplant, Fennel, Garlic, Kale, Kohlrabi, Leeks, Lettuces, Mushrooms, Okra, Onions, Peas, Bell Peppers, Chili Peppers, Potatoes, Radish, Rhubarb, Shallots, Spinach, Squash, Tomatoes.

Holidays:

4th of July - Many of my patients get off track on summer weekends, especially three-day holiday weekends where we celebrate all weekend long. Lowering the calorie density of your food can really help. Calorie density is basically the amount of calories in a given weight of food, so, for example a cup of lettuce has low calorie density while a cup of butter has a high calorie density. Using calorie density to your advantage is one of the absolute keys to long-term weight loss. This concept can be a very valuable tool when navigating food-filled barbeques like the 4th of July. Here are secrets to navigating those barbeques without derailing your diet:

1. **Slim down your sides** – What's a barbeque without chips and dip? If you can't live without them, enjoy yours the smart way. Mix equal parts salsa or pico de gallo and guacamole to cut calories almost in half without shrinking your serving size. You can also slash calories by making dips with low-fat or non-fat sour cream or yogurt instead of the full fat varieties. You'll never notice the difference flavor wise, I promise. Serving these with baked or popped chips instead of fried chips lets you enjoy in moderation minus the guilt. Skip the potato salad and opt for whole-wheat pasta salad made with a light vinaigrette and loaded with veggies to bring down the calorie density. Or try our skinny and delicious Golden Couscous Salad.

2. **Build a better burger** – Mix equal parts lean ground beef or turkey with ground mushrooms to instantly cut calories in half. Just make sure to steer clear of cheese or mayo which bumps up the calorie density right back to

where you started. Instead, try spicy mustard or chipotle sauce for flavor without boosting the calorie density. Serve your burger on a whole-wheat bun (it's packed with filling fiber) and top it with romaine lettuce instead of iceberg for an extra nutrition boost. Or try our tasty, satisfying Green Chili Turkey Burger.

3. Dilute your drinks – Unsweetened, calorie-free beverages are best, especially if you'll be sipping all day long. If you really want lemonade, juice, or white wine, mix yours with equal parts sparkling water to save calories without feeling like you're missing out.

4. Lower the density of your dessert – You can always enjoy fresh seasonal fruit with a little whipped topping for dessert, but sometimes that just doesn't cut it. Instead of limiting yourself to a tiny brownie or half a cookie, why not bake your own lower calorie dessert? Try adding canned pumpkin (it's packed with fiber and a great source of vitamins A, C and K) or applesauce to your favorite baked goodie recipe instead of oil. You'll keep calories under control without having to eat mini portions.

Summer Travel

Travel can be an incredible time to relax, visit new places - and try new foods. But just because you're on vacation doesn't mean that your diet has to be on vacation too. When you're on the road it's not realistic to expect that you'll eat perfectly. After all, sampling the local eats is half the fun. By making a few smarter choices, and staying active, you'll be surprised how you can enjoy your vacation and keep those numbers on the scale in check. Here's how:

1. Pack healthy snacks – whether you're travelling by plane, train or automobile, make sure you have plenty of healthy snacks on hand. My favorites include protein rich energy bars, fresh fruit, single serving size bags of nuts, turkey jerky, string cheese, hard boiled eggs or even a half a peanut butter and jelly sandwich on whole-wheat bread. Stash these in your travel bag and you'll be a lot less likely to be tempted by junk food at the airport or mini mart.

2. Plan ahead - call your hotel and find out if they serve breakfast or have a mini-fridge. If they don't serve breakfast, bring along instant oatmeal for a quick and healthy breakfast. If they have a mini-fridge, you're in luck! Find a local market and stock the fridge with healthy snacks like low-fat yogurt, single serve low-fat cottage cheese, carrots and hummus, turkey slices and sparkling water. That way, when you get back to your room after a long day of fun, you can have a good-for-you nosh before dinner – one of the best preventive measures to make sure you don't show up to dinner famished. To save calories - and money -have a yogurt topped with high fiber cereal and fruit for breakfast instead of going out every day.

3. Stock the freezer before you leave - buy a few healthy frozen meals so that when you get home, exhausted, after a wonderful vacation you'll have a day or two of healthy eating options at your fingertips. You'll be a lot less likely to order greasy Chinese take-out or pizza.

Chapter Five: Fall

September, October, Early November

Overview: Right now, your schedule is probably fairly normal again (if there is such a thing!) and you're ready to buckle down until the holiday season begins. This is a good time to shape up your diet by cutting back a little on fruit and starchy carbs and also get organized again when it comes to exercise.

The only major holiday in September is Labor Day, so this month shouldn't be too much of a challenge. In early October you may have the three-day weekend, Columbus Day off, but this shouldn't be too much of a problem. The major diet derailer of the season is Halloween, followed by the first week of November, when you have to deal with a house filled with leftover candy.

With the temperature dropping, you'll likely be craving warm, comforting food. We'll come to the rescue with lots of ideas for savory, satisfying stick-to-your ribs soups and meals.

Exercise: Even if you haven't been great about workouts over the summer, build a new fitness routine for the fall. Try to include at least 45 minutes of cardio four to five times a week. If you don't have much time during the week, squeeze in at least 20 minutes twice a week and exercise for at least an hour on both weekend days. If you don't belong to a gym, now may be the time to invest in a new exercise DVD to help you get excited about working out again. With the holidays right around the corner, now is the time to challenge yourself physically to kick weight loss into high gear.

Behavior: Instead of beating yourself up for how you may have strayed from your diet over the summer, flip to the end of the book again and repeat the exercise that you did in March. Write down several things you did well over the summer (I'm sure there were a few) as well as at least three goals you'd like to reach before Thanksgiving.

If you're having trouble getting back into a healthy routine, take it one step at a time. First, focus on getting your diet back on track for a week or two. Then slowly ease into the exercise component. Weigh yourself every 10 days instead of once a week, as weight loss may be slower at this point. I don't want you to get discouraged chasing a number on the scale. If you find that the scale is driving you crazy, don't weight yourself for a while. Instead, pick a tight fitting pair of pants and try them on weekly instead. Sometimes the stress of not seeing numbers on the scale move can actually backfire. If you find this happening, do your best to focus on eating better and exercising more instead.

Be sure to keep a food journal to trouble shoot, if necessary. I find that with many of my patients, extra calories tend to creep back in the longer they are on a 'diet'. If you find that this is the case, take a good luck at your food journal to see where the extra calories are sneaking in and then do damage control by cleaning things up as much as you can.

Seasonal Produce:

SEPTEMBER
Fruits:
Apples, Avocados, Blackberries, Dates, Figs, Grapefruit, Grapes, Kiwi, Lemons, Melons, Nectarines, Peaches, Pears, Plums, Pomegranate, Quince, Raspberries, Strawberries.

Vegetables:
Artichokes, Arugula, Beans, Beets, Bok Choy, Broccoli, Brussels Sprouts, Cabbage, Cauliflower, Celery, Chard, Collards, Corn, Cucumbers, Endive, Eggplant, Garlic, Kale, Leeks, Lettuces, Mushrooms, Okra, Olives, Onions, Peas, Bell Peppers, Chili Peppers, Potatoes, Radish, Rhubarb, Shallots, Spinach, Squash, Tomatoes.

OCTOBER
Fruits:
Apples, Avocados, Dates, Figs, Grapefruit, Grapes, Kiwi, Kumquats , Lemons, Limes, Melons, Nectarines, Oranges, Peaches, Pears, Plums, Pomegranates, Quince, Raspberries, Strawberries.

Vegetables:
Artichokes, Arugula, Beans, Beets, Bok Choy, Broccoli, Brussels Sprouts, Cabbage, Cauliflower, Celery, Chard, Collards, Corn, Cucumbers, Endive, Eggplant, Garlic, Kale, Kohlrabi, Leeks, Lettuces, Mushrooms, Okra, Olives, Onions, Parsnip, Peas, , Bell Peppers, Chili Peppers, Potatoes, Radish, Rhubarb, Shallots, Spinach, Squash, Tomatoes.

NOVEMBER
Fruits:
Apples, Avocados, Pears, Dates, Figs, Grapes, Guava, Lemons, Kiwi, Limes, Mandarins, Orange, Pomegranate, Raspberries, Strawberries.

Vegetables:
Artichokes, Arugula, Beans, Beets, Bok Choy, Broccoli, Brussels Sprouts, Cabbage, Carrots, Cauliflower, Celeriac, Chard, Celery, Collards, Corn, Cucumber, Endive, Fennel, Garlic, Ginger, Kale, Kohlrabi, Leeks, Lettuce, Mushrooms, Okra, Onions, Olives, Parsnip, Peas, Potatoes, Bell Peppers, Chili Peppers, Rhubarb, Shallots, Spinach, Sprouts, Squash, Turnips, Yams.

Holidays

Early September: Labor Day – the last barbeque of summer time. Referring back to 4th of July strategies can help you start the Fall season off on the right foot. Consider serving our Fall Grilled Chicken Pesto Wraps or Fall Asian Chicken Salad at your labor day BBQ for two healthy, yet hearty options.

1st Half of October: Columbus Day - this isn't usually a big eating day, but it is a day off for many of us. Take advantage of the extra time and beautiful fall weather to do something active outdoors like a going for a long walk or hike, playing a game of tag football with the family, or loading up the bikes and heading out of town for a long bike ride in the countryside.

October 31 Halloween - there's no doubt about it, Halloween is one of the most challenging holidays if you're watching your weight. Not only is candy everywhere, it seems like you're surrounded by loads of leftover candy (at home and in the office) for at least a week afterward. Last year, I was shocked to find three candy bowls at my dentist's office the Monday after Halloween. But that doesn't mean you're destined to succumb to temptation. Instead try these tips that I've collected over the years:

1. **Don't buy candy that you like.** One of my former patients made this suggestion and I thought it was an ingenious idea! If you love peanut butter cups, don't buy them. Otherwise you'll have to face the leftovers every day until you run out (translation: eat them all). That's just asking for problems.
2. **Keep candy hidden** in an upper cabinet until Halloween. I've talked about this before – out of sight means out of mind. Why constantly tempt yourself with a big bowl of candy on the counter?

3. Arm yourself at the office. If candy is everywhere, stock up on mini lollipops, mints and sugar free gum to keep your mouth occupied and away from the mini chocolate buffet in the break room.

4. Donate leftovers. Many of my patients donated their leftover candy to the troops overseas this year, a win-win situation.

5. Think Outside the (Candy) Box. Halloween doesn't just have to be about candy. Dip apples in a light caramel sauce for a tasty treat or try low fat kettle corn instead. Both are lower in calories plus they provide a healthy dose of fiber to help fill you up.

2nd Week of November: Veterans Day -
again, not a big eating day, but an ideal opportunity to sneak in an extra 30 minutes or more of exercise.

Why not take part of the day to prep healthy meals for the rest of the week? That way you'll make as much healthy eating progress as possible before Thanksgiving which is just a couple of weeks away.

Chapter Six: Early Winter

Late November, December

Overview: Early winter is when things start to get really challenging in the diet department. November began with too much candy and ends with what is probably the biggest eating day of the year: Thanksgiving. Before you know it, December is here and the holiday chaos really begins. Between stressful holiday shopping, office cocktail parties, travel, and family holiday dinners, extra calories from food and drinks seem pretty much unavoidable. I tell all of my patients that if they can simply maintain their weight between Thanksgiving through New Years it's a huge victory. While you may be able to shed a few pounds in early November, the reality for most of us is that it's just too hard to completely control calories once December hits. Your mission: Aim to maintain. If you can still manage to lose, all the better for next year.

Exercise: Whatever you do, please don't abandon your workouts completely, even if you have to cut them in half (or less). You really need to schedule workouts into your day, even if your schedule is hectic. In addition, try to take any opportunity you can to squeeze in 10-minute bouts of extra exercise throughout the day to keep burning those calories.

Behavior: It's essential that you don't turn off your diet plan this month. If you do, the result could be a serious – and very discouraging – weight gain. Research shows that most normal weight people usually gain only a pound or two over the holidays, but overweight people often gain five to ten pounds. I don't expect you to eat perfectly this month – there's just too much temptation. But you can make better choices and trade- offs that will allow you to have your cake and eat it too, at least some of the time.

Get on the scale once a week to keep yourself from veering too far off track. Many of my patients avoid the scale completely when they aren't paying attention to their diet and ignore the fact that their favorite pair of pants is getting tighter every day. It might also be useful to keep a food journal this month so you can try to balance out the frequent splurges with lower calorie meals.

Take a moment right now to do the following exercise: Briefly describe how you'll feel if you get on the scale January 1 and you are at the same weight that you were December 1.

_____

_____

_____

_____

Here are some easy strategies to keep you from tipping the scales this month.

1. **Never go to a cocktail or dinner party famished.** Eat a small (100 to 150 calorie) protein and fiber rich snack (like ½ cup of whole grain cereal with non-fat or 1% milk or non-fat Greek yogurt with ½ cup of fresh berries) and drink a

large glass of water before heading out the door to help you minimize indulgences and resist temptation more easily.

2. Set the stage for success. At cocktail parties try not to stand near the buffet and face away from it if you can. Eat off an appetizer plate, if possible, and drink out of tall thin glasses if you have the option. These three strategies will help you eat and drink less effortlessly.

3. Watch the alcohol. Alcohol can wreak havoc on your willpower when it comes to making smart food choices. Plus, the calories add up quickly, especially when sugary cocktails or eggnog are involved. To minimize the effect of alcohol (and keep your willpower intact), nibble on something with a little bit of fat before you drink (like a few nuts or a small piece of cheese).

4. Look before you load. Look over the entire buffet before you fill your plate so that you can decide ahead of time what you are going to splurge on as well as what will fill you up for fewer calories.

5. Squeeze in exercise and up the intensity. Once the holidays hit, you probably won't have time for your full workout. If not, try to squeeze in mini workouts (10 to 15 minutes) whenever you can and up the intensity.

6. Use the two-thirds rule. Load two-thirds of your plate with healthier options like lean protein and vegetables and use the remaining third for indulgences that you rarely eat but really enjoy. Be sure to focus on treats rather than foods that you can eat anytime. Skip the chips and dip or cheese and crackers and go for small servings of foods you can only get around the holidays.

7. Think trade-offs. Trade-offs are always important, but even more so over the holidays. Having a cocktail? Skip the dessert (or just have one bite). On the flip side, if you feel you absolutely must have dessert, pass on the alcohol or limit yourself to one glass and then switch to sparkling water with lime.

8. Send leftovers packing. If you're entertaining, send guests home with a care package of leftovers (especially desserts) to minimize temptation on your end. If your husband or kids can't bear to part with all the leftovers, at least make sure those tempting goodies are out of sight, either in the cabinet or the back
of the fridge.

9. Wear tight fitting clothes. Seriously! This constant (and somewhat uncomfortable) reminder that you're eating too much can be a huge help.

10. Eat water-rich foods when you're at home. They'll keep you full for fewer calories. Whip up our recipes like Black Bean Soup with Avocado Crème or Balsamic Turkey Cutlets with Swiss Chard. They'll keep you full and satisfied for surprisingly few calories.

Seasonal Produce:

DECEMBER
Fruits:
Avocados, Dates, Grapefruit, Grapes, Guavas, Kumquats, Lemons, Limes, Mandarins, Pomegranates, Tangerines.

Vegetables:
Artichokes, Beans, Beets, Bok Choy, Broccoli, Brussels Sprouts, Cabbage, Carrots, Cauliflower, Chard, Celery, Collards, Endive, Fennel, Garlic, Kale, Kohlrabi, Leeks, Lettuce, Mushrooms, Onions,

Parsnip, , Bell Peppers, Chili Peppers, Potatoes, Radish, Spinach, Squash, Yams.

Holidays:

Late November: Thanksgiving - this day has the dubious distinction of being the biggest eating day of the year. If you can, I suggest that you really watch your diet in the days leading up to Thanksgiving to make room for the extra calories you'll probably be eating. If you're travelling, re-read the travel tips from July.

On Thanksgiving Day, start the day with a simple, low carb breakfast like our Chicken Apple Sausage Frittata. If you need a morning snack, choose from the 100-calorie snack list only. For lunch, toss up a big salad with protein like our Asian Chicken Salad. If possible, about 30 minutes before dinner, have a cup or two of vegetable soup to take the edge off of your appetite. Then when it's time for your Thanksgiving meal, follow my general tips for holiday eating.

If you really want to stay on track, here are two roadmaps (one from my co-author Karen and the other from me, which is a bit more indulgent!) for a Thanksgiving plate that won't sink your diet.

- **Karen's Thanksgiving Dinner:** 2 slices of white meat turkey, 1 cup green beans with 1 teaspoon olive oil, ½ baked sweet potato and 2 tablespoons cranberry sauce. For dessert, opt for a small slice of pumpkin pie and cut off the thick piece of crust at the end (that's where most of the calories are).

- **Dr. Melina's Thanksgiving Dinner:** (I always try to work out extra hard before dinner to make room for a little extra indulgence on my plate). 2 slices of white meat turkey, 1 cup of green beans with 1 tbsp. slivered almonds,

½ cup candied sweet potatoes (my cousin is a chef in New Orleans and makes a sweet potato dish that's to die for), ½ cup stuffing, sliver of pecan pie with the end crust cut off (admission: I'm not a huge fan of pumpkin pie).

If you're hosting Turkey Day, the last thing you want is for one day of indulgence to turn into four. So try to give away as many of the tempting leftovers as possible. For exercise, plan a short but high intensity workout in the morning (it can be longer if you have time). If possible, take a 20 to 30 minute (or longer) walk after dinner or do something active inside with your family (like cranking up some music and having a mini dance party).

Late December: Hanukkah, Christmas Eve and Day, Kwanzaa - Follow my earlier holiday eating tips and focus on the company, not just the food. Try to enjoy everything in moderation and don't beat yourself up if you get a little off track.

December 31: New Year's Eve - If you're drinking, don't drink on an empty stomach. Food is key for slowing down the absorption of alcohol, and keeping your willpower intact. Alternate a glass of sparkling or flat water with each alcoholic drink you have. If you're also eating dinner, you may want to limit your intake of starchy carbs to make room for those additional alcohol calories. Happy New Year's!

January 1 – Final Thoughts

As the calendar year comes to a close and a new year begins, I hope that you've made significant progress working towards your diet and fitness goals. Even if you didn't accomplish everything you hoped, keep in mind that weight loss is a long term process. You probably didn't gain all of your excess weight in a year, so it's only natural that it may take a little longer to lose it. That's okay! When you lose weight slowly you're much more likely to maintain that weight loss – for good.

By continuing to use the strategies, recipes and tips outlined in this book, you can continue to work towards your goals. Weight loss isn't easy, and maintaining weight loss is almost as challenging. It requires constant mindfulness and a commitment to leading a healthier lifestyle. You don't have to be perfect every day. There will be days when that giant chocolate chip cookie is just too tempting. Just try to stay on the right path most of the time.

When it comes to keeping those pounds off, exercise is a critical part of the equation. So continue to challenge yourself and find activities that you enjoy.
I can assure you that your continued pursuit of a healthier lifestyle is definitely worth every bit of the year-round effort in helping you to achieve optimal health and live your best life.

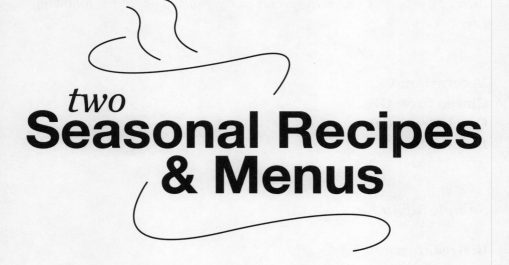

two Seasonal Recipes & Menus

If you have special diet restrictions, many of these recipes are vegetarian, low carb, gluten free or can be made in a hurry. Please note that the gluten free recipes call for gluten free versions of all ingredients listed. For those of you with special restrictions, look for the following icons:

Vegetarian: V
Gluten Free: GF
Quick Prep: QP
Low Carb: LC

Sample Menu Key:

B: Breakfast
S: Snack
L: Lunch
D: Dinner

Winter Recipes & Sample Menu

chapter seven

Chicken Apple Sausage Frittata

Peanut Butter & Jelly Oatmeal

Maple Pear Ricotta Toast

Curried Chickpea Burgers

Tilapia Provencal

Tomato Basil Ricotta Pizza

Penne with Brussels Sprouts & Bacon

No Guilt Nachos

Chicken Tortilla Soup

Portobello Steak

Roast Chicken Spinach Salad

White Bean Vegetable Soup

Oven Baked Chicken Milanese

Chocolate Fondue

Winter Sample Menu Day

B: Maple Pear Ricotta Toast
S: 2 tbsp. or 100 calorie pack of nuts
L: Chicken Tortilla Soup
S: 2 Mandarin oranges + 1 string cheese
D: Oven Baked Chicken Milanese
1 five-ounce glass of wine (optional)

Winter Sample Menu Day – Lower Carb

B: Chicken Apple Sausage Frittata
S: 1 cup non-fat Greek yogurt (plain or vanilla)
L: Roast Chicken Spinach Salad
S: 1 apple + 1 tbsp. peanut butter
D: Tilapia Provencal
Dessert – 1 ounce of dark chocolate

Winter Sample Menu Day – Vegetarian

B: Peanut Butter & Jelly Oatmeal
S: 1 string cheese + 1 tangerine
L: White Bean Vegetable Soup
S: 14 baby carrots + ¼ cup hummus
D: Tomato Basil Ricotta Pizza
Dessert: ½ sliced apple dipped in ¼ cup non-fat
Greek yogurt with ½ tsp sugar

Breakfast

Chicken Apple Sausage Frittata (QP, LC)

Ingredients: Serves 1

1 teaspoon unsalted butter
2 tablespoons chopped onion
1/2 chicken apple sausage link, cut into ¼-inch dice
1 egg
3 egg whites
Dash salt
Dash pepper

Directions:
1.   Preheat broiler.
2.   In a medium skillet, melt butter over medium-low heat.
3.   Add onions and sauté 2 minutes. Add sausage and sauté for 2 additional minutes.
4.   Scramble egg, egg whites, salt and pepper. Pour into pan and reduce heat to low. Cook until eggs just begin to set, about 3 to minutes.
5.   Place pan under broiler for 1-2 additional minutes until top is completely set. Remove from skillet and serve.

Nutrition stats: 243 cals, 24g protein, 5g carbs, 1g fiber, 14g fat (6g sat)

Peanut Butter & Jelly Oatmeal (QP, V)

Ingredients: Serves 1

½ cup rolled oats
1 cup water
Pinch salt
1 teaspoon sugar
2 teaspoons chunky peanut butter
2 teaspoons all-fruit preserves

Directions:
1. Cook oats in water with salt according to package directions.
2. Stir in sugar.
3. Top with peanut butter and preserves. Stir briefly and serve.

Nutrition stats: 270 calories, 9g protein, 40g carbs, 5g fiber,
8g fat (1g sat)

Maple Pear Ricotta Toast (V, QP)

Ingredients: Serves 1

1/3 cup non-fat ricotta cheese
½ teaspoon maple syrup
Pinch cinnamon
2 slices whole-wheat bread, toasted
½ pear, cored and sliced

Directions:
1. In a small bowl, mix ricotta, syrup and cinnamon together
   until thoroughly combined.
2. Spread ricotta mixture on toast. Top with sliced pear.

Nutrition stats: 268 calories, 13g protein, 51g carbs, 7g fiber, 2g fat
(0g sat)

Lunch And Dinner

Curried Chickpea Burgers (V)

Ingredients: Serves 2

1 egg white
1/3 cup quick cooking oats
1/3 cup chopped red onion
1/2 teaspoon curry powder
1/4 teaspoon cumin
Large pinch corriander
Large pinch cinnamon
1/4 teaspoon salt
Pinch pepper
1 cup no salt added canned chickpeas, rinsed and drained
Non-stick cooking spray
3 tablespoons non-fat Greek yogurt
1 tablespoon mango chutney
2 6-inch whole-wheat pitas, sliced in half
1/4 cucumber, sliced
2 thin slices red onion, cut in half
Cilantro sprigs, if desired

Directions:
1. Place chickpeas, egg white, oats, onion, spices, salt and pepper in a food processor. Pulse until smooth, about 2-3 minutes.
2. Form into 4 patties.
3. Spray a griddle or large pan with cooking spray. Heat over medium heat. Add patties and cook 8 minutes, turning halfway Remove from heat.
4. While burgers are cooking, whisk chutney into Greek yogurt.
5. Place 1 burger into each pita half. Stuff each half with cucumber, onion and cilantro. Top each pita half with 1 tablespoon yogurt chutney sauce.

Nutrition stats: 399 calories, 18g protein, 73g carbs, 12g fiber, 5g fat (0g sat)

Tilapia Provencal (GF)

Ingredients: Serves 2

2 6-ounce tilapia filets
14.5-ounce can diced tomatoes
1 clove garlic, chopped
1 tablespoon capers, drained
1 tablespoon fresh lemon juice
2 teaspoons lemon zest
2 teaspoons olive oil
Pinch salt
Pinch pepper
Pinch red pepper flakes
½ teaspoon dried oregano
1 cup cooked brown rice

Directions:
1. Preheat oven to 375F.
2. Pla ce tilapia in a 13 x 9 baking dish.
3. In a medium bowl, combine tomatoes, garlic, capers, lemon
    juice, lemon zest, olive oil, salt, pepper, red pepper and oregano.
    Pour over tilapia and cover tightly with foil. Bake for 20 minutes
    or until fish flakes easily.
4. Remove from oven and serve over brown rice.

Nutrition stats: 360 calories, 38g protein, 33g carbs, 4g fiber, 8g fat (2g sat)

Tomato Basil Ricotta Pizza (V, QP)

Ingredients: Serves 2

¼ cup pizza sauce
½ ready-made 12-inch whole-wheat pizza crust
3 tablespoons non-fat ricotta cheese
1 ounce sliced mozzarella cheese, cubed
2 fresh basil leaves, torn

Directions:
1. Preheat oven to 400F.
2. Spread sauce on pizza crust.
3. Top with dollops of ricotta cheese and mozzarella pieces.
4. Bake for 8-10 minutes, until cheese is melted.
5. Remove from oven. Sprinkle with basil, slice in half and serve.

Nutrition stats: 344 calories, 18g protein, 55g carbs, 10g fiber, 7g fat (3g sat)

Penne with Brussels Sprouts and Bacon

Ingredients: Serves 2

4 ounces multi grain penne
1 tablespoon olive oil
1 cup onion, cut into 1-inch dice
1-½ cups Brussels sprouts, quartered
¼ teaspoon salt
Pinch pepper
1 cup low-sodium chicken broth
1 tablespoon fresh lemon zest
1 slice bacon, cooked and crumbled
3 tablespoons grated Parmesan cheese

Directions:
1. Cook pasta according to package directions. Drain and set aside.
2. While pasta is cooking, heat olive oil in a large skillet over
medium-low heat. Add onion and sauté for 2 minutes. Add Brussels sprouts and sauté 7 minutes.
3. Season Brussels sprouts with salt and pepper. Reduce heat to low. Add chicken broth and sauté 5 additional minutes.
4. Stir in lemon zest. Remove from heat. Add cooked pasta, bacon and Parmesan. Toss well and serve.

Nutrition stats: 396 calories, 19g protein, 53g carbs, 8g fiber, 13g fat (3g sat)

No Guilt Nachos

Ingredients: Serves 2

4 6-inch corn tortillas, cut into sixths
Olive oil cooking spray
¼ teaspoon chili powder, divided
¼ teaspoon cumin, divided
¼ teaspoon garlic powder, divided
½ teaspoon Kosher salt, divided
1 medium tomato, diced
1/3 cup chopped Vidallia onion
1 tablespoon fresh lime juice
2 tablespoons chopped fresh cilantro, plus additional for garnish
1 cup no salt added canned pinto beans, rinsed and drained
½ cup reduced-fat shredded cheddar cheese
½ cup non-fat Greek yogurt

Directions:
1. Preheat oven to 350F.
2. Arrange tortilla pieces on a baking sheet. Spray tops with cooking spray. Sprinkle with half of chili powder, cumin, garlic and salt. Reserve remaining spices.
3. Bake for 15 min. Remove from oven & set aside
4. In a medium bowl combine remaining spices, salt, tomato, onion, lime juice and cilantro. Set aside.
5. Warm beans in microwave for 1 minute. Stir beans into tomato mixture.
6. Arrange tortilla chips on a large oven-proof plate. Sprinkle with cheese and heat in oven, until cheese is just melted, about 3 to 5 minutes.
7. Remove from oven. Top with tomato-bean mixture, Greek yogurt and additional cilantro if desired.

Nutrition stats: 363 calories, 19g protein, 50g carbs, 6g fiber, 8g fat (3g sat)

Chicken Tortilla Soup (GF)

Ingredients: Serves 2

2 teaspoons olive oil
1 cup Vidallia onion, cut into 1-inch dice
1 clove garlic, minced
3 cups low-sodium chicken broth
14.5-ounce can diced tomatoes
2 tablespoons canned diced chili peppers
1 cup shredded skinless rotisserie chicken breast
¼ teaspoon cumin
Pinch red pepper flakes
¼ teaspoon salt
2 tablespoons fresh lime juice
2 tablespoons chopped fresh cilantro
3 6" corn tortillas, cut into ½-inch strips

Directions:

1. Heat oil over medium-low heat in a large stock pot. Add onion and sauté 2 minutes. Add garlic and sauté 1 additional minute.

2. Add chicken broth, tomatoes, chili peppers, chicken, cumin, red pepper and salt. Bring to boil. Reduce heat to low. Simmer 20 minutes.

3. Remove from heat. Stir in lime juice, cilantro and tortilla strips.

Nutrition stats: 401 calories, 33g protein, 43g carbs, 5g fiber, 11g fat (2g sat)

Portobello Steak

Ingredients: Serves 2

2 teaspoons olive oil
2 portobello mushrooms, cut into ½-inch slices
1 clove garlic, minced
½ teaspoon kosher salt, divided
2 pinches black pepper
¼ cup low-sodium chicken or beef broth
1 tablespoon Worcestershire sauce
1 tablespoon balsamic vinegar
1 tablespoon tomato paste
¼ teaspoon garlic powder
6 ounces lean flank steak
Non-stick cooking spray
2 tablespoons reduced-fat sour cream

Directions:
1. Bake potato in a 400F oven until soft, about 1 hour.
2. While potato is baking, heat olive oil in a large skillet over medium heat. Add mushrooms and sauté until soft, about 5 minutes.
3. Add garlic and sauté 1 additional minute. Season with ¼ teaspoon salt and 1 pinch pepper. Reduce heat to low.
4. Whisk together broth, Worcestershire sauce, vinegar, and tomato paste. Add to pan and cook 30 seconds. Remove from heat.
5. Season steak with garlic powder and remaining salt and pepper.
6. Spray a large skillet or grill pan with non-stick cooking spray. Heat over medium-high heat. Add steak and cook 10 minutes, turning halfway. Remove from heat and slice.
7. Toss steak with mushrooms. Divide between 2 plates and serve alongside 1/2 baked potato topped with 1 tablespoon sour cream.

Nutrition stats: 372 calories, 26g protein, 41g carbs, 5g fiber, 11g fat (3g sat)

Roast Chicken Spinach Salad (QP)

Ingredients: Serves 2

6 cups baby spinach
1 cup shredded skinless rotisserie chicken
1 cup grape tomatoes, halved
¼ cup thinly sliced red onion
4 tablespoons honey mustard salad dressing
14 whole-wheat pita chips, crumbled

Directions:
1. In a large salad bowl, toss spinach, chicken, tomatoes and onions with salad dressing.
2. Divide between 2 plates. Top with pita chips.

Nutrition stats: 370 calories, 27g protein, 28g carbs, 6g fiber, 17g fat (2g sat)

White Bean Vegetable Soup (GF)

Ingredients: Serves 2

2 teaspoons olive oil
1-ounce slice Canadian bacon, cut into 1/4-inch dice
1 cup chopped onion
1 carrot, cut into 1/4-inch dice
¼ fennel bulb, cut into 1/4-inch dice
¼ teaspoon salt
Large pinch pepper
1 clove garlic, minced
3 cups low-sodium chicken broth
15.5-ounce can no salt added cannellini beans, rinsed and drained
1 cup chopped canned tomatoes
½ teaspoon finely chopped fresh rosemary
Pinch crushed red pepper flakes
3 tablespoons grated Parmesan cheese

Directions:
1.   In a large stock pot, heat olive oil over medium-low heat. Add Canadian bacon, onion, carrot and fennel and season with salt and pepper. Sauté 4 minutes. Add garlic and sauté 1 additional minute.
2.   Add chicken broth, beans, tomatoes, rosemary and red pepper flakes. Bring to a low boil and lower heat to a simmer. Simmer for 20 minutes.
3.   Remove from heat. Add Parmesan cheese and mix well.

Nutrition stats: 371 calories, 22g protein, 51g carbs, 13g fiber, 10g fat (2g sat)

Oven Baked Chicken Milanese

Ingredients: Serves 2

1 egg
2 6-ounce boneless, skinless chicken breast halves
½ cup seasoned breadcrumbs
Non-stick cooking spray
2 cups chopped arugula
4 large basil leaves, roughly chopped
2 medium tomatoes, diced
½ chopped red onion
Large pinch salt
Large pinch pepper
1 tablespoon balsamic vinegar
2 teaspoons extra virgin olive oil

Directions:
1. Preheat oven to 400F.
2. Scramble egg in shallow bowl. Add chicken to coat. Remove chicken and dredge in breadcrumbs.
3. Place chicken in a baking dish sprayed with non-stick cooking spray. Bake for 30-35 minutes, or until internal temperature reaches 165F. Remove from oven.
4. While chicken is cooking, toss together arugula, basil, tomato, onion, salt, pepper, balsamic vinegar and olive oil together in a medium bowl.
5. Divide salad between 2 serving plates. Top each plate with 1 piece of chicken.

Nutrition stats: 414 calories, 44g protein, 27g carbs, 3g fiber, 14g fat (3g sat)

Chocolate Fondue (QP,V)

Ingredients: Serves 2

3 tablespoons semisweet chocolate chips
1 banana, sliced

Directions:
1. Place chocolate chips in a small microwave-safe bowl.
Microwave for 1½ to 2½ minutes, until chocolate chips
arenearly melted. Stir well until chocolate chips are
completely
melted and mixture is smooth and creamy.
2. Serve with banana slices for dipping.

Nutrition stats: 158 calories, 2g protein, 27g carbs, 3g fiber,
6g fat (4g sat)

Spring Recipes & Sample Menu

chapter eight

Strawberry Stuffed French Toast

Smoked Salmon Chive Bagel Thin

Egg Whites Rancheros

Edamame Burgers

Teriyaki Chicken Kebabs

Pasta with Spring Vegetables

Chicken Corn Cheddar Quesadillas

Thai Peanut Noodles

Orange Glazed Pork Chops over

Bok Choy

Sesame Tuna Over Baby Spinach

Spaghetti with White Beans

Arugula & Feta

Chili Lime Chicken

Shrimp Fajitas

Spring Sample Menu Day

B: Egg White Rancheros
S: 1 cup strawberries + ½ cup low-fat cottage cheese
L: Chicken Corn Cheddar Quesadillas
S: 2-3 celery sticks + 1 tbsp. peanut butter
D: Spaghetti with White Beans Arugula & Feta
1 five-ounce glass of wine (optional)

Spring Sample Lower Carb Day

B: Smoked Salmon Chive Bagel Thin
S: 1 string cheese + 6-8 strawberries
L: Sesame Tuna Over Baby Spinach
S: ¼ cup nuts + small orange
D: Orange Glazed Pork Chops over Bok Choy

Spring Sample Vegetarian Day

B: Strawberry Stuffed French Toast
S: 2 tbsp. of nuts + mandarin orange
L: Pasta with Spring Vegetables
S: 2-3 whole grain crackers + ¼ cup hummus
D: Edamame Burgers
Dessert: ½ cup non-fat vanilla yogurt + 1 graham cracker crumbled

Breakfast

Strawberry Stuffed French Toast (QP, V)

Ingredients: Serves 1

½ cup sliced strawberries
½ teaspoon sugar
1 large egg
1 egg white
2 slices whole-wheat bread
1 teaspoon unsalted butter

Directions:
1. Place strawberries in a small microwave-safe bowl. Sprinkle with sugar and toss. Microwave until slightly bubbling, about
45 seconds. Remove from microwave and set aside.
2. In a small bowl, scramble egg and egg white together.
3. Top 1 slice bread with 1 tablespoon of strawberry mixture. Reserve remaining mixture. Press remaining slice of bread firmly on top of bottom piece to make a sandwich.
4. Heat butter in a medium skillet over medium-low heat.
5. Dip French toast into egg mixture, coating both sides thoroughly. Place in skillet and cook for 4 to 6 minutes, until golden brown, turning halfway.
6. Remove from skillet and top with remaining strawberry sauce.

Nutrition stats: 296 calories, 16g protein, 38g carbs, 6g fiber, 11g fat (4g sat)

Smoked Salmon Chive Bagel Thin (QP)

Ingredients: Serves 1

1 whole-wheat bagel thin
1 tablespoon whipped cream cheese
3 ounces smoked salmon
2 slices tomato
1 thin slice red onion, if desired
1 tablespoon minced chives

Directions:
1. Toast bagel thin.
2. Spread half of bagel thin with cream cheese. Top with smoked salmon, tomato and onion. Sprinkle with chives.
3. Top with remaining half bagel thin.

Nutrition stats: 257 calories, 23g protein, 27g carbs, 6g fiber, 8g fat (3g sat)

Egg Whites Rancheros (V, QP)

Ingredients: Serves 1

1 teaspoon unsalted butter
4 egg whites
Pinch salt
Pinch pepper
1 6-inch corn tortilla
¼ cup no sodium added black beans, rinsed and drained
½ cup diced tomatoes
2 tablespoons tomatillo salsa
2 tablespoons non-fat plain Greek yogurt
1 tablespoon chopped fresh cilantro

Directions:

1. Heat butter in small skillet over medium heat.
2. Scramble egg whites with salt and pepper.
3. Add eggs to skillet and cook until firm, about 2 to 3 minutes.
4. Arrange tortilla on plate. Top with cooked egg whites, black beans, tomatoes, salsa, Greek yogurt and cilantro.

Nutrition stats: 261 calories, 22g protein, 30g carbs, 5g fiber, 5g fat (2g sat)

Lunch And Dinner

Edamame Burgers (V)

Ingredients: Serves 2

3/4 cup frozen edamame, thawed
1/3 cup chopped onion
1/3 cup panko
1 egg white
½ teaspoon minced fresh ginger
2 teaspoons low-sodium soy sauce
Pinch pepper
Non-stick cooking spray
2 whole-wheat deli or sandwich flats
4 teaspoons reduced-fat canola oil mayonnaise
¼ teaspoon prepared wasabi or wasabi paste, or to taste
½ cup baby spinach leaves
2 thin slices onion

Directions:
In a food processor pulse edamame, onion, panko, egg white, ginger, soy sauce and pepper until smooth, about 2 to 3 minutes. Divide and form into 2 tightly packed burger patties.

1. Spray a large sauté pan or griddle with non-stick spray. Heat over medium-low heat. Add burgers and cook for 10 to 12 minutes, carefully flipping halfway. Remove from heat.
2. While burgers are cooking whisk together mayonnaise and wasabi.
3. Spread wasabi mayonnaise on deli flats. Layer with burgers, spinach and onions.

Nutrition stats: 284 calories, 17g protein, 43g carbs, 7g fiber, 6g fat (0 sat)

Teriyaki Chicken Kebabs

Ingredients: Serves 2

2 tablespoons low-sodium soy sauce
1 tablespoon rice wine vinegar
1 teaspoon Dijon mustard
2 teaspoons canola oil
8 ounces skinless, boneless chicken breast, cut into 1-inch cubes
1 cup pineapple, cut into 1-inch chunks
2 scallions, cut into 1-inch pieces
Pinch salt
Pinch pepper
1 cup cooked brown rice

Directions:
1.   In a small bowl, whisk together soy sauce, rice vinegar, mustard and canola oil.
2.   Place chicken, pineapple and scallions in a 1-gallon zip top plastic bag and add marinade. Seal tightly and marinate in refrigerator for at least 2 hours or overnight.
3.   Drain marinade from chicken pineapple mixture and discard. Alternately thread chicken, pineapple and scallions on 2 metal skewers. Sprinkle with salt and pepper. Broil or grill for 8 to 10 minutes, turning halfway.
4.   Remove from heat and serve each skewer with ½ cup cooked brown rice.

Nutrition stats: 339 cals, 28g protein, 36g carbs, 3g fiber, 9g fat (1g sat)

Pasta with Spring Vegetables (V)

Ingredients: Serves 2

1 cup asparagus, cut into 1-inch pieces
4 ounces whole-wheat rotini pasta
1 tablespoon olive oil
½ cup chopped Vidalia onion
2 cloves garlic, thinly sliced
½ cup low-sodium chicken or vegetable broth
¾ cup frozen peas, thawed
¼ teaspoon salt
Pinch pepper
3 tablespoons grated Parmesan cheese
2 teaspoons minced chives
4 basil leaves, chopped

Directions:
1.   Bring a large pot of water to a boil. Add asparagus and cook for 2 minutes. Remove from heat. Remove asparagus with a slotted spoon and set aside.
2.   Return water to heat and bring to a boil. Add pasta and cook according to package directions. Drain and set aside.
3.   In a large sauté pan, heat olive oil over medium-low heat. Add onion and sauté for 2 minutes. Add garlic and sauté 1 additional minute.
4.   Reduce heat to low. Add broth, peas, asparagus, salt and pepper. Cook for 2 minutes. Remove from heat.
5.   Toss hot pasta with Parmesan cheese. Add to sautéed vegetables and toss again.
6.   Divide between two serving plates and top with chives and basil.

Nutrition stats: 383 cals, 15g protein, 57g carbs, 10g fiber, 11g fat (2g sat)

Chicken Corn Cheddar Quesadillas (GF, QP)

Ingredients: Serves 2

1 teaspoon olive oil
1/3 cup chopped onion
2/3 cup frozen corn, thawed
½ cup skinless rotisserie chicken breast, cut into ½-inch dice
Pinch pepper
Pinch salt
1 scallion, thinly sliced
Non-stick cooking spray
4 6-inch corn tortillas
½ cup reduced-fat shredded sharp cheddar cheese
4 tablespoons salsa

Directions:
1. In a medium sauté pan, heat olive oil over medium-low heat. Add onion and sauté for 2 minutes. Add corn, chicken, salt and pepper. Sauté 2 additional minutes. Stir in scallion. Remove from heat.
2. Spray a large sauté pan or griddle with non-stick cooking spray.
Heat over medium heat.
3. Divide cheese in half. Spread each half over 2 of the tortillas.
Top each with half of corn-chicken mixture and top with remaining tortilla.
4. Heat quesadillas in pan or griddle for 5 to 6 minutes, turning halfway. Remove from heat.
5. Slice each quesadilla in sixths and serve with salsa.

Nutrition stats: 355 calories, 22g protein, 43g carbs, 4g fiber, 11g fat (4g sat)

Thai Peanut Noodles (V)

Ingredients: Serves 2

4 ounces linguine
2 tablespoons peanut butter
1 ½ tablespoons low-sodium soy sauce
2 teaspoons brown sugar
1 tablespoon fresh lime juice
1 tablespoon rice wine vinegar
1 pinch red pepper flakes, or to taste
½ cup cooked edamame
½ cup shredded carrots
¼ cucumber quartered, and sliced
2 teaspoons chopped fresh mint

Directions:
1.   Cook pasta to package directions. Drain and set aside.
2.   While pasta is cooking, whisk together peanut butter, soy sauce, brown sugar, lime juice, rice vinegar and red pepper flakes.
3.   Place cooked linguine in a large bowl with edamame, carrots and cucumber. Drizzle with dressing and toss well.
4.   Top with mint and serve.

Nutrition stats: 392 cals, 18g pro, 60g carbs, 4g fiber, 10g fat (2g sat)

Orange Glazed Pork Chops over Bok Choy (GF, LC)

Ingredients: Serves 2

3 teaspoons canola oil, divided
1 head bok choy, roughly chopped
2 5-ounce boneless pork chops
2 pinches salt
2 pinches pepper
2 tablespoons sherry
¼ cup orange juice
¼ cup low-sodium chicken broth
1 tablespoon all fruit orange marmalade

Directions:
1.   Heat 1 teaspoon canola oil in a large sauté pan over medium heat. Add bok choy and sauté until just wilted, about 5 minutes.
Remove from heat and set aside.
2.   Season pork chops with salt and pepper.
3.   Heat 2 teaspoons canola oil in a large sauté pan over medium heat. Add pork chops, turning after 5 minutes.
Cook 3 additional minutes. Reduce heat to low. Add sherry, orange juice and chicken broth.
4.   Cook 2 additional minutes or until pork reaches an internal temperature of 145F. Remove pork from pan and set aside.
5.   Whisk marmalade into pan juices until thoroughly combined.
6.   Divide bok choy between two plates. Top each plate with one pork chop. Spoon half of pan juices over each pork chop.

Nutrition stats: 363 calories, 38g protein, 16g carbs, 4g fiber, 15g fat (3g sat)

Sesame Tuna Over Baby Spinach (QP, LC)

Ingredients: Serves 2

2 6-ounce tuna filets
Pinch salt
Pinch pepper
Non-stick cooking spray
2 tablespoons low-sodium soy sauce
1 tablespoon rice wine vinegar
2 teaspoons canola oil
1 teaspoon sesame oil
½ teaspoon minced fresh ginger
½ teaspoon honey
4 cups baby spinach

Directions:
1. Season tuna with salt and pepper.
2. Spray a non-stick grill pan with cooking spray. Heat over medium-high heat. Add tuna and cook 4 minutes for rare or 6 minutes for medium, turning halfway. Remove from heat.
3. While tuna is cooking, whisk together soy sauce, rice vinegar, canola oil, sesame oil, ginger and honey.
4. Place spinach in a large salad bowl. Drizzle with 3 tablespoons soy vinaigrette. Divide spinach between 2 plates. Top each with 1 tuna fillet and drizzle with remaining vinaigrette.

Nutrition stats: 348 cals, 42g pro, 9g carbs, 2g fiber, 16g fat (3g sat)

Spaghetti with White Beans Arugula & Feta (QP, V)

Ingredients: Serves 2

4 ounces dry whole-wheat spaghetti
1 tablespoon olive oil
2 cloves garlic, thinly sliced
1 cup no sodium added canned cannellini beans, rinsed and drained
½ cup low-sodium chicken or vegetable broth
½ teaspoon Dijon mustard
¼ teaspoon salt
Pinch pepper
4 cups chopped arugula
2 tablespoons feta cheese crumbles

Directions:
1. Prepare spaghetti according to package directions. Drain and set aside.
2. While pasta is cooking, heat oil in a large sauté pan over medium-low heat. Add garlic and sauté 1 minute.
3. Reduce heat to low. Add beans, broth, mustard, salt and pepper.
Stir well to combine and sauté 2 minutes. Add arugula and sauté until just wilted, about 5 minutes.
4. Add spaghetti to saucepan and toss well. Top with feta and serve.

Nutrition stats: 400 cals, 18g protein, 63g carbs, 13g fiber, 11g fat (2g sat)

Chili Lime Chicken (GF, LC)

Ingredients: Serves 2

2 5-ounce boneless, skinless chicken breast halves
2 pinches salt, divided
2 pinches pepper, divided
1 pinch garlic powder
1/2 teaspoon plus 1 pinch chili powder, divided
4 teaspoons canola oil
4 tablespoons fresh lime juice
1 teaspoon honey
1 tablespoon chopped fresh cilantro
4 cups shredded romaine lettuce
1/2 cucumber, thinly sliced
2 radishes, thinly sliced

Directions:
1.   Season chicken with 1 pinch each salt, pepper, garlic powder and chili powder.
2.   Heat 1 teaspoon canola oil in a medium skillet over medium heat. Add chicken and cook 10 to 12 minutes, or until chicken reaches an internal temperature of 165F, turning halfway. Remove from heat and set aside.
3.   While chicken is cooking whisk together lime juice, honey, cilantro and remaining canola oil, salt, pepper and chili powder.
4.   Toss romaine, cucumber and radishes in a large salad bowl. Drizzle with half of dressing and toss well.
5.   Divide salad between 2 plates. Top each with 1 piece of chicken and drizzle with remaining dressing.

Nutrition stats: 292 cals, 32g pro, 11g carbs, 3g fiber, 13g fat (2g sat)

Shrimp Fajitas (QP)

Ingredients: Serves 2

2 teaspoons canola oil
1 yellow bell pepper, sliced
½ large Vidalia onion, sliced
10 large shrimp, peeled and deveined
Pinch salt
Pinch pepper
Pinch garlic powder
2/5 avocado, diced
2 8-inch whole-wheat tortillas
¼ cup salsa verde

Directions:
1. Heat canola oil in a large sauté pan over medium heat. Add
yellow pepper and onion. Saute for 5 minutes, until soft.
Remove from pan and set aside.
2. Season shrimp with salt, pepper and garlic powder. Add to
pan and sauté over medium heat for 5 minutes, turning
half way. Remove from heat.
3. Layer tortillas with half of shrimp, sautéed vegetables and
avocado. Serve with salsa.

Nutrition stats: 298 cals, 11g protein, 36g carbs, 6g fiber,
13g fat (2g sat)

Summer Recipes & Sample Menu

chapter nine

Apricot Orange Waffles

Raspberry Peach Smoothie

Honey Fig Breakfast Sundae

Grilled Chicken BLT Salad

Fish Tacos with Cilantro Lime Slaw

Green Chili Turkey Burgers

Golden Couscous Salad

Seared Steak and Blue Cheese Salad

Spaghetti with Fresh Tomatoes,
Corn, Shrimp and Basil

BBQ Chicken Pizza with Pineapple

Seared Scallop Nectarine Salad

Grilled Chicken Gyros

Curried Quinoa with Chickpeas
and Apricots

Summer Sample Menu Day

B: Apricot Orange Waffles
S: 2 celery sticks + 1 tbsp. peanut butter
L: Seared Steak and Blue Cheese Salad
S: 1 cup non-fat Greek yogurt topped with 1/2 cup fresh berries
D: BBQ Chicken Pizza with Pineapple
Dessert: 1 no sugar added frozen fruit bar

Summer Sample Lower Carb Day

B: Honey Fig Breakfast Sunday
S: 2 tbsp. nuts + 1 apricot
L: Seared Scallop Nectarine Salad
S: 1 cup cherries + 1 string cheese
D: Grilled Chicken BLT Salad
One white wine spritzer (optional)

Summer Sample Vegetarian Day

B: Raspberry Peach Smoothie
S: 100 calorie pack of nuts (or 2 tbsp.)
L: Golden Couscous Salad
S: 1/2 cup low fat cottage cheese + 1 plum
D: Curried Quinoa with Chickpeas and Apricots
Dessert: 1 mini s'more

Breakfast

Apricot Orange Waffles (QP, V)

Ingredients: Serves 1

2 teaspoons orange marmalade all fruit spread
¼ cup non-fat ricotta cheese
2 whole grain waffles, toasted
2 apricots, sliced

Directions:
1.   Whisk fruit spread into ricotta.
2.   Spread half of ricotta mixture onto each toasted waffle.
3.   Top each waffle with 1 sliced apricot. If desired, make a sandwich by placing on waffle on top of the other with fruit in the middle.

Nutrition stats: 297 cals, 10g pro, 47g carbs, 4g fiber, 7g fat

Raspberry Peach Smoothie (GF, V, QP)

Ingredients: Serves 1

¾ cup frozen peaches, roughly diced
¾ cup frozen raspberries
1 cup non-fat plain Greek yogurt
½ cup orange juice
1 teaspoon agave nectar

Directions:
1. Combine all ingredients in blender.
2. Blend on high speed until mixture is completely smooth, about 3-4 minutes.

Nutrition stats: 272 cals, 22g protein, 49g carbs, 5g fiber, 0g fat (0g sat)

Honey Fig Breakfast Sundae (GF, QP, V)

Ingredients: Serves 1

1 cup 1% cottage cheese
2 medium figs, quartered
1 tablespoon slivered almonds
½ teaspoon honey

Directions:
1. Scoop cottage cheese into small serving bowl.
2. Top with figs and almonds.
3. Drizzle with honey and serve.

Nutrition stats: 281 calories, 30g protein, 29g carbs, 4g fiber, 5g fat (2g sat)

Lunch And Dinner

Grilled Chicken BLT Salad (LC)

Ingredients: Serves 2

1 6-ounce boneless, skinless chicken breast half
Pinch salt
Pinch pepper
Pinch garlic powder
6 cups shredded romaine lettuce
1 cup grape tomatoes, halved
4 tablespoons Italian vinaigrette
1 slice cooked bacon, crumbled

Directions:
1. Preheat grill or broiler.
2. Season chicken with salt, pepper and garlic powder.
3. Grill or broil chicken 8 to 10 minutes (or until chicken reaches an internal temperature of 165F), turning halfway. Remove from heat and slice.
4. In a large salad bowl toss lettuce, tomatoes and chicken with vinaigrette.
5. Divide between 2 plates. Top with crumbled bacon.

Nutrition stats: 397 cals, 43g protein, 21g carbs, 6g fiber, 16g fat (2g sat)

Fish Tacos with Cilantro Lime Slaw (GF)

Ingredients: Serves 2

Cilantro Lime Slaw:
1-1/2 tablespoons fresh lime juice
1 tablespoon rice wine vinegar
1 tablespoon canola oil
1 teaspoon sugar
1/4 teaspoon salt
1 large pinch pepper
1-1/2 teaspoons lime zest
3 cups shredded cabbage or coleslaw mix

Fish tacos:
8 ounces firm white fish such as barramundi, cod or or tilapia
1/4 teaspoon chili powder
1/4 teaspoon cumin
Large pinch salt
Large pinch pepper
Non-stick cooking spray
4 6-inch corn tortillas

Directions:
1.   In a medium bowl, whisk together lime juice, rice vinegar, canola oil, sugar, salt, pepper and lime zest. Add shredded cabbage. Toss well and set aside.
2.   Season fish with chili powder, cumin, salt and pepper.
3.   Spray a griddle pan or large sauté pan with non-stick spray and heat over medium-high heat. Add fish and cook 6 to 8 minutes (or until fish flakes easily), turning halfway.
4.   Divide fish among tortillas. Top with coleslaw and serve.

Nutrition stats: 355 cals, 27g protein, 37g carbs, 5g fiber, 12g fat (1g sat)

Green Chili Turkey Burgers

Ingredients: Serves 2

1 teaspoon canola oil
½ cup chopped onion
6 ounces ground turkey (at least 93% lean)
1-½ tablespoons canned diced green chili peppers
2 teaspoons Worcestershire sauce
1 tablespoon ketchup
Large pinch salt
Large pinch pepper
Non-stick cooking spray
2 whole-wheat hamburger buns
2 slices tomato
2 slices red onion
2 tablespoons barbeque sauce

Directions:
1. In a small sauté pan, heat canola oil over medium-low heat. Add onions and sauté for 2 minutes. Set aside.
2. In a medium bowl, combine turkey, chili peppers, Worcestershire sauce, ketchup, cooked onions, salt and pepper. Mix well and form into 2 patties.
3. Spray a large sauté pan or griddle pan with non-stick spray.
Heat over medium heat. Add turkey burgers and cook for 10 minutes (until burgers reach an internal temperature of 165F), turning halfway. Remove from heat.
4. Serve burgers on whole-wheat hamburger buns with tomato and onion slices and barbeque sauce.

Nutrition stats: 322 cals, 22g protein, 38g carbs, 5g fiber, 10g fat (2g sat)

Golden Couscous Salad

Ingredients: Serves 2

2 teaspoons olive oil
2 tablespoons minced shallots
1 cup low-sodium chicken or vegetable broth
¼ teaspoon salt
Pinch pepper
½ cup whole-wheat couscous
2 tablespoons golden raisins
1 tablespoon lemon zest
1/3 cup grated carrots
1 tablespoon sliced almonds
1 cup skinless rotisserie chicken breast, cut into 1/2-inch dice
1 tablespoon chopped mint

Directions:
1.   Heat olive oil in a medium saucepan over medium-low heat. Add shallots and sauté for 2 minutes.
2.   Add broth, salt and pepper and bring to a boil. Remove from heat.
3.   Stir in couscous and raisins and cover for 10 minutes. Uncover and fluff with fork.
4.   Add lemon zest, carrots, almonds, chicken and mint. Toss well to combine all ingredients. Serve warm or chilled.

Nutrition stats: 400 cals, 31g protein, 50g carbs, 8g fiber, 9g fat (2g sat)

Seared Steak and Blue Cheese Salad (LC)

Ingredients: Serves 2

6 ounces lean flank steak
Pinch salt
Pinch pepper
Pinch garlic powder
2 teaspoons canola oil
½ medium red onion, sliced
6 cups baby spinach
1 large tomato, cut into 1/8ths
4 tablespoons balsamic vinaigrette
2 tablespoons blue cheese crumbles

Directions:
1.   Season steak with salt, pepper and garlic powder.
2.   Heat canola oil in a medium sauté pan over medium heat. Add onions and sauté until just softened, about 3 minutes.
3.   Remove onions from pan and set aside. Increase heat to medium-high. Add steak and cook for 8 to 10 minutes, turning
halfway. Remove from heat.
4.   In a large salad bowl, toss cooked onions, spinach and tomato with balsamic vinaigrette. Divide between 2 plates.
5.   Slice steak and layer on top of salad. Sprinkle with blue cheese crumbles.

Nutrition stats: 315 cals, 24g protein, 21g carbs, 5g fiber, 16g fat (4g sat)

Spaghetti with Fresh Tomatoes, Corn, Shrimp & Basil

Ingredients: Serves 2

4 ounces whole-wheat spaghetti
12 large shrimp, cleaned and deveined
2 pinches salt, divided
2 pinches pepper, divided
Pinch garlic powder
1 tablespoon olive oil
1 ear corn, kernels removed
1 clove garlic, sliced
¼ cup white wine
1/3 cup low-sodium chicken or vegetable broth
1 large tomato, cut into ¼-inch dice
2 tablespoons chopped fresh basil
2 tablespoons Feta cheese crumbles

Directions:

1. Cook pasta in a large pot of boiling water according to directions. Drain & set aside.
2. While pasta is cooking, season shrimp with 1 pinch each salt, pepper and garlic powder.
3. Heat olive oil in a large sauté pan over medium heat. Add corn & sauté for 5 minutes. Reduce heat to medium-low & add garlic. Sauté 1 additional minute. Remove corn from pan & set aside.
4. Return pan to stove and heat over medium heat. Add shrimp and cook 5 minutes, turning halfway. Remove shrimp from pan and set aside.
5. Return pan to stove and heat over medium-low heat. Add wine and broth and cook 2 minutes, scraping up brown bits from bottom of pan. Add tomato and cooked corn, cooking 1 additional minute. Season with remaining salt and pepper. Remove from heat.
6. Add pasta and shrimp to pan and toss well.
7. Divide between 2 plates. Top with basil & Feta.

Nutrition Stats: 395 calories, 18g protein, 58g carbs, 9g fiber, 10g fat (2g sat)

BBQ Chicken Pizza with Pineapple (QP)

Ingredients: Serves 2

½ cup shredded skinless rotisserie chicken breast
2 tablespoons barbeque sauce
½ ready-made 12-inch whole-wheat pizza crust
½ cup pineapple chunks
1 scallion, sliced
¼ cup shredded reduced-fat cheddar cheese

Directions:
1. Preheat oven to 400F.
2. Toss chicken with barbeque sauce.
3. Top pizza crust with chicken, pineapple and scallion. Sprinkle with cheese.
4. Bake for 8 to 10 minutes, until cheese is melted. Remove from oven and serve.

Nutrition stats: 400 calories, 27g protein, 63g carbs, 10g fiber, 6g fat (2g sat)

Seared Scallop Nectarine Salad (GF)

Ingredients: Serves 2

12 sea scallops
Pinch salt
Pinch pepper
1 tablespoon plus 1 teaspoon extra virgin olive oil, divided
2 tablespoons orange juice
1 teaspoon Dijon mustard
½ teaspoon honey
6 cups butter lettuce
2 nectarines, sliced

Directions:
1. Season scallops with salt and pepper.
2. Heat 1 teaspoon of olive oil in a large sauté pan over medium
high heat. Add scallops and cook for 3 minutes, turning
halfway. Remove from heat and set aside.
3. In a small bowl, whisk together remaining olive oil, orange
juice, mustard and honey.
4. In a large bowl, toss lettuce and nectarine with dressing.
Divide between 2 plates. Top each with 6 scallops.

Nutrition Stats: 239 calories, 14g protein, 25g carbs, 4g fiber, 11g fat (2g sat)

Grilled Chicken Gyros

Ingredients: Serves 2

1 6-ounce boneless, skinless chicken breast half
2 tablespoons Italian vinaigrette, divided
1 cup shredded romaine lettuce
4 Kalamata olives, sliced
4 slices red onion
1 medium tomato, cut into ¼-inch dice
¼ cucumber, cut into ¼-inch dice
2 6-inch whole-wheat pitas, sliced in half
½ cup non-fat Greek yogurt

Directions:
1. Marinate chicken in 1 tablespoon salad dressing in refrigerator for 1 hour or overnight.
2. Preheat grill or broiler.
3. Grill or broil chicken 8 to 10 minutes (until chicken reaches an internal temperature of 165F), turning halfway. Remove from heat and slice.
4. In a medium bowl, toss romaine, olives, onion, tomatoes, cucumber and cooked chicken.
5. Stuff salad into pita halves. Top each half with 2 tablespoons
Greek yogurt.

Nutrition Stats: 393 calories, 31g protein, 47g carbs, 7g fiber, 10g fat (2g sat)

Curried Quinoa with Chickpeas and Apricots (V, GF)

Ingredients: Serves 2

1 teaspoon olive oil
¼ cup chopped onion
1 cup low-sodium chicken or vegetable broth
½ cup dry quinoa
¼ teaspoon curry powder
Large pinch cinnamon
Pinch salt
1 teaspoon orange zest
¼ cup chopped dried apricots
1 cup no salt added chickpeas, rinsed and drained

Directions:

1.   Heat olive oil in a medium stockpot over medium-low heat. Add onion and sauté for 2 minutes.

2.   Add broth. Raise heat and bring to a boil. Add quinoa, curry,
cinnamon and salt. Cover and reduce heat to low. Cook for 10 minutes.

3.   Uncover and stir in orange zest and apricots. Cover and continue to cook for 5 additional minutes.

4.   Remove from heat and add chickpeas. Toss well, cover and let stand for 5 minutes before serving.

Nutrition stats: 366 cals, 15g protein, 64g carbs, 10g fiber, 6g fat (1g sat)

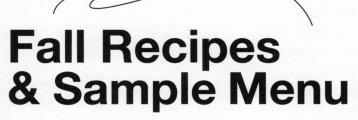

Fall Recipes & Sample Menu
chapter ten

Fall Sample Menu Day

B: Almond Butter and Banana Quesadilla
S: 1 cup non-fat Greek yogurt
L: Asian Chicken Salad
S: 2 tbsp. nuts + pear
D: Lemon Shrimp Over Couscous
1 five-ounce glass of white wine (optional)
Summer Sample Menu Day

Fall Sample Lower Carb Day

B: Cheddar Egg Muffin
S: 1 small apple + 1 tbsp. peanut butter
L: Tuna, Grape and Arugula Salad
S: 14 baby carrots + ¼ cup hummus
D: Balsamic Turkey Cutlets with Swiss Chard
Dessert: 1 ounce of dark chocolate

Fall Sample Vegetarian Day

B: Apple Pomegranate Breakfast Parfait
S: ¼ cup of nuts
L: Black Bean Soup with Avocado Crème
S: 2-3 whole grain crackers + 1 slice reduced fat cheese
D: Pumpkin Polenta
Dessert: ½ cup melon + 2 tbsp. non-fat vanilla yogurt

Breakfast

Almond Butter and Banana Quesadilla (QP, V)

Ingredients: Serves 1

Non-stick cooking spray
1 8-inch whole-wheat tortilla
1 tablespoon almond butter
½ banana, sliced

Directions:
1. Spray a medium skillet with cooking spray. Heat over medium low heat.
2. Cut tortilla in half. Spread 1 half with almond butter. Top with banana slices. Top with remaining half tortilla.
3. Place in skillet, banana side down. Heat for 2 minutes. Flip and heat 1 additional minute. Remove from skillet and serve.

Nutrition stats: 288 cals, 8g protein, 38g carbs, 6g fiber, 13g fat (2g sat)

Apple Pomegranate Breakfast Parfait (V, GF)

Ingredients: Serves 1

1 6-ounce container non-fat plain Greek yogurt
1 tablespoon pomegranate juice
1 teaspoon agave nectar
Dash nutmeg
1 apple, cored and diced
2 tablespoons pomegranate seeds
1 tablespoon chopped walnuts

Directions:
1. Spoon yogurt into small serving bowl or container. Whisk in pomegranate juice, agave nectar and nutmeg.
2. Top with apple, pomegranate seeds & walnuts.

Nutrition stats: 265 calories, 17g protein, 41g carbs, 6g fiber, 5g fat (1g sat)

Cheddar Egg Muffin (QP, V)

Ingredients: Serves 1

1 egg
Dash salt
Dash pepper
Non-stick cooking spray
1 sprouted grain English muffin, toasted
1 tablespoon reduced-fat shredded Cheddar cheese
1 slice tomato

Directions:

1. Scramble egg with salt and pepper. Pour into a small ramekin that has been sprayed with non-stick cooking spray.
2. Microwave for 30 seconds. Remove from microwave. Sprinkle with cheddar cheese and microwave for 10 additional seconds or until eggs are firm.
3. Remove from ramekin and place on half of toasted English muffin.
4. Top with tomato and remaining half English muffin.

Nutrition stats: 254 calories, 16g protein, 32g carbs, 6g fiber, 7g fat (2g sat)

Lunch And Dinner

Pumpkin Polenta (GF, V)

Ingredients: Serves 2

1 1/3 cups low-sodium chicken broth
1 cup non-fat milk
2/3 cup quick cooking polenta
½ cup canned pureed pumpkin
½ teaspoon maple syrup
2 large pinches cinnamon
Pinch nutmeg
Pinch black pepper
3 tablespoons grated Parmesan cheese

Directions:
1. Bring chicken broth and milk to a boil in a medium saucepan.
2. Add polenta and stir well. Reduce heat to low. Simmer 5-10 minutes, until smooth and creamy, stirring frequently.
3. Stir in pumpkin, maple syrup, cinnamon, nutmeg and pepper. Cook 2 additional minutes.
4. Stir in Parmesan and serve.

Nutrition stats: 341 calories, 16g protein, 54g carbs, 6g fiber, 7g fat (3g sat)

Mini Meatball Soup

Ingredients: Serves 2

2 ounces elbow macaroni
4 ounces 95% lean ground beef
1 egg white
2 tablespoons seasoned breadcrumbs
3 tablespoons grated Parmesan cheese, divided
Large pinch salt
2 large pinches pepper, divided
1 clove minced garlic, divided
2 teaspoons olive oil
½ cup chopped onion
3 cups low-sodium chicken broth
1 cup diced canned tomatoes
1 tablespoon tomato paste
¼ teaspoon dried oregano
2 cups baby spinach, roughly chopped

Directions:

1. Cook macaroni according to package directions. Drain and set aside.
2. In a medium bowl, combine ground beef, egg white, breadcrumbs, 1 tablespoon Parmesan, salt, 1 large pinch pepper, and ½ of garlic. Form into 8 small meatballs. Set aside.
3. In a large stockpot, heat olive oil over medium-low heat. Add onion and sauté for 2 minutes. Add remaining garlic and sauté 1 additional minute.
4. Add chicken broth, tomatoes, tomato paste, oregano and remaining pepper. Bring to a boil. Reduce heat to low and simmer for 10 minutes. Add meatballs. Cover and simmer 12 additional minutes.
5. Remove from heat. Stir in macaroni, remaining Parmesan and spinach and serve.

Nutrition stats: 373 calories, 28g protein, 41g carbs, 4g fiber, 11g fat (3g sat)

Tuna, Grape and Arugula Salad (QP)

Ingredients: Serves 2

6 cups chopped arugula
5-ounce can water packed tuna, drained
1 cup red grapes, halved
1 apple, cored and cut into ½-inch dice
¼ cup thinly sliced fennel
4 tablespoons balsamic vinaigrette
2 tablespoons sunflower seeds

Directions:
1. In a large salad bowl, toss arugula, tuna, grapes, apple, fennel and vinaigrette.
2. Divide between 2 plates, top with sunflower seeds and serve.

Nutrition stats: 342 cals, 19g protein, 33g carbs, 5g fiber, 15g fat (1g sat)

Black Bean Soup with Avocado Crème (GF, V)

Ingredients: Serves 2

2 teaspoons olive oil
½ cup chopped onion
1 clove garlic, minced
15.5-ounce can no sodium added black beans, rinsed and drained
1 cup chopped canned tomatoes
2 cups low-sodium vegetable or chicken broth
½ teaspoon cumin
¼ to ½ teaspoon chili powder
¼ teaspoon salt
Large pinch black pepper
¼ cup non-fat Greek yogurt
¼ avocado
½ teaspoon lime zest
1 teaspoon fresh lime juice

Directions:
1.   Heat olive oil in a large stockpot over medium-low heat. Add onions and sauté for 2 minutes. Add garlic and sauté 1 additional minute.
2.   Add black beans, tomatoes, broth, spices, salt and pepper. Bring to a boil and reduce heat to low. Simmer uncovered for 20 minutes. Remove from heat.
3.   While soup is cooking puree Greek yogurt, avocado, lime zest and lime juice in a blender 2-3 minutes, until smooth. Set aside.
4.   Allow soup to cool slightly until it is lukewarm. Transfer to a blender or food processor. Puree until smooth, 2-4 minutes. Return to pot, mix well and reheat.
5.   Divide soup between two bowls. Top each bowl with half of avocado crème.

Nutrition stats: 315 cals, 17g protein, 43 g carbs, 12g fiber, 8g fat (1g sat)

Grilled Chicken Pesto Wrap (QP)

Ingredients: Serves 2

Non-stick cooking spray
2 thinly sliced 4-ounce boneless, skinless chicken breast cutlets
Pinch salt
Pinch pepper
Pinch garlic powder
2 8-inch whole-wheat tortillas
4 teaspoons pesto
2 1-ounce slices jarred, roast peppers, drained
½ cup arugula leaves

Directions:

1. Spray a large sauté pan or grill pan with non-stick spray. Heat pan over medium heat.
2. Season chicken with salt, pepper and garlic powder.
3. Add chicken to pan and cook 6-8 minutes, until cooked through, turning halfway. Remove from heat. Allow to cool slightly. Cut into ½-inch slices.
4. Spread each tortilla with 2 teaspoons pesto. Top each with half of chicken, roast peppers and arugula. Roll into wrap, cut in half and serve.

Nutrition stats: 326 cals, 30g pro, 25g carbs, 4g fiber, 12g fat (3g sat)

Skinny Chicken Parmigiana

Ingredients: Serves 2

4 ounces dry angel hair pasta
2 thinly sliced 4-ounce boneless, skinless chicken breast cutlets
Pinch salt
Pinch pepper
Pinch garlic powder
2 teaspoons olive oil
1/2 cup marinara sauce
1/4 cup reduced-fat shredded mozzarella cheese
2 fresh basil leaves, roughly chopped

Directions:
1.   Prepare pasta according to package directions. Drain and set aside.
2.   While pasta is cooking, season chicken with salt, pepper and garlic powder.
3.   Preheat broiler.
4.   Heat oil in a medium skillet over medium heat. Add chicken and cook 6 to 8 minutes, until cooked through, turning halfway.
5.   Remove chicken from skillet and place on baking sheet. Top each cutlet with 1/4 cup marinara sauce and 2 tablespoons cheese. Place under boiler for 1 to 2 minutes, until cheese is melted. Remove from broiler and top each cutlet with half of basil.
6.   Divide angel hair between 2 plates and top each with one chicken cutlet.

Nutrition stats: 395 calories, 24g protein, 47g carbs, 3g fiber, 12g fat (3g sat)

Balsamic Turkey Cutlets with Swiss Chard (GF, LC)

Ingredients: Serves 2

4 teaspoons canola oil, divided
8 cups Swiss Chard, stems removed and roughly chopped
3 tablespoons low-sodium chicken or vegetable broth
2 tablespoons balsamic vinegar, divided
2 tablespoons golden raisins
Dash nutmeg
2 pinches salt, divided
2 pinches pepper, divided
2 5-ounce turkey breast cutlets
1 clove garlic, thinly sliced

Directions:
1.   Heat 2 teaspoons canola oil in a large sauté pan over medium heat. Add Swiss chard, broth, 1 tablespoon balsamic vinegar, raisins, nutmeg, 1 pinch salt and 1 pinch pepper. Sauté until wilted, about 5 minutes. Set aside.
2.   Season turkey cutlets with remaining salt and pepper.
3.   Heat remaining oil in a large sauté pan over medium heat. Add turkey and cook 6 minutes, turning halfway, until turkey is golden brown and cooked through.
4.   Add garlic to pan and stir briefly for 30 seconds. Remove pan from heat and add remaining balsamic vinegar. Stir well until turkey cutlets are coated with vinegar.
5.   Divide Swiss chard between 2 plates. Top each with 1 turkey cutlet and serve.

Nutrition stats: 311 cals, 38g protein, 17g carbs, 3g fiber, 10g fat (1g sat)

BBQ Chicken and Sweet Potatoes

Ingredients: Serves 2

2 6-ounce sweet potatoes
2 5-ounce skinless, boneless chicken breast halves
Pinch salt
Pinch pepper
2 teaspoons canola oil
¼ cup barbeque sauce

Directions:
1.   Bake sweet potato in a 425F oven, until soft, about 1 hour. Remove and set aside.
2.   Season chicken with salt and pepper.
3.   Heat canola oil in a large skillet over medium heat. Add chicken. Cook 10 to 12 minutes, or until chicken reaches an internal temperature of 165F, turning halfway.
4.   Remove chicken from pan and brush with barbeque sauce.   Serve each chicken breast with 1 baked sweet potato.

Nutrition stats: 358 cals, 33g protein, 35g carbs, 4g fiber, 9g fat (1g sat)

Lemon Shrimp Over Couscous

Ingredients: Serves 2

½ cup whole-wheat couscous
1 cup low-sodium chicken or vegetable broth
12 large shrimp, peeled and deveined
2 pinches salt, divided
2 pinches pepper, divided
1 tablespoon olive oil
¼ cup white wine
2 tablespoons fresh lemon juice
2 teaspoons lemon zest
1 tablespoon capers, drained

Directions:
1.   Cook couscous in broth according to package directions. Set aside.
2.   While couscous is steaming, season shrimp with 1 pinch each salt and pepper.
3.   Heat olive oil in a large sauté pan over medium heat. Add shrimp and cook 5 minutes, turning halfway.
Remove from pan.
4.   Add white wine to pan and cook 1 minute, scraping up any brown bits on bottom of pan. Reduce heat to low. Add lemon juice, lemon zest, capers, and remaining salt and pepper.
Return shrimp to pan and stir well to combine.
Remove from heat.
5.   Divide couscous between 2 plates. Serve shrimp over couscous.

Nutrition stats: 297 cals, 14g pro, 40g carbs, 6g fiber, 8g fat (1g sat)

Asian Chicken Salad (LC, QP)

Ingredients: Serves 2

6 cups shredded romaine lettuce
1 cup shredded skinless rotisserie chicken
1 apple, quartered, cored, and thinly sliced
¼ cup sliced drained water chestnuts
½ cup shredded carrots
4 tablespoons Asian vinaigrette

Directions:
1. In a large salad bowl, toss romaine, chicken, apple, water chestnuts, carrots and vinaigrette.
2. Toss well, divide between 2 plates and serve.

Nutrition stats: 336 cals, 24g protein, 29g carbs, 7g fiber, 14g fat (2g sat)

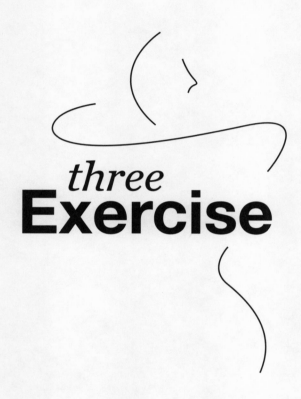

three
Exercise

Introduction

Exercise is crucial for losing weight and maintaining that weight loss. Circuit training is one of the most effective and time efficient ways to exercise. It offers both strength and cardiovascular benefits. These calorie-burning workouts will challenge your entire body with a combination of cardio, lower body, upper body and core exercises. Each circuit includes nine exercises: six strength-based exercises and three cardiovascular exercises.

Level 1 (If you're new to working out/haven't exercised in over 6 months):

The Circuit includes: 6 strength exercises* + 3 cardiovascular exercises
2 lower body exercises – 1 from Category A + 1 from Category B
2 upper body exercises – 1 from Category C + 1 from Category D
2 abdominal/core exercises from Category E
3 cardiovascular exercises from Category F
* Choose the modified versions of the exercises when available.

Exercise Order:
1 CIRCUIT = Category A > Rest > Category C > Rest > Category F > Rest > Category B > Rest > Category D > Rest > Category F > Rest > Category E > Rest > Category E > Rest > Category F > Rest (Repeat circuit)**

**Complete one circuit for a shorter/less intense workout. For faster results and a more challenging workout, repeat the circuit 3 times.

Exercise Duration:
Strength exercises (Category A-E) = 30 seconds
Cardiovascular exercises (Ctategory F) = 1-2 minutes

Rest = 10-20 seconds between exercises
One circuit = 7 – 12 minutes (depending on cardiovascular
& rest time)

Level 2 (Workout at least twice/week for 6 months):

The Circuit includes: 6 strength exercises* + 3 cardiovascular
exercises
2 lower body exercises – 1 from Category A + 1 from Category B
2 upper body exercises – 1 from Category C + 1 from Category D
2 abdominal/core exercises from Category E
3 cardiovascular exercises from Category F
* Choose the advanced versions of the exercises when available.

Exercise Order:
1 CIRCUIT = Category A > Category C > Category F >
Category B > Rest > Category D > Rest > Category F > Rest
> Category E > Rest > Category E > Rest > Category F (Repeat
circuit)**
**Complete one circuit for a shorter/less intense workout. For
faster results & a more challenging workout, repeat the circuit
3 times.

Exercise Duration:
Strength exercises (Category A-E) = 60 seconds
Cardiovascular exercises (Category F) = 2-3 minutes
Rest = Minimal
One circuit = 12 – 15 minutes (depending on cardiovascular time)

Equipment:
Light Pair of Weights: Women = 3 to 5 lbs each; Men = 8 to 10 lbs
each Heavy Pair of Weights: Women = 10 to 12 lbs each; Men =
15 to 20 lbs each
Resistance Band: Women = Light or medium resistance; Men =
Heavy resistance.

The Workout Program

Chart Key: (see below for full descriptions)
Cir = Circuit
CA = Cardio
HIIT = High Intensity Interval Training
P = Pyramid training
AR = Active Rest
R = Rest

MON	TUE	WED	THURS	FRI	SAT	SUN
Cir	CA, HIIT or P	Cir	AR	Cir	CA, HIIT or P	R

The Warm-up: Warming up is essential to any workout. Warm up exercises prepare your muscles and joints for more intense activity by increasing circulation and body temperature, as well as preventing injuries. Always make sure to warm up before you stretch.

Recommended warm-up:

1) March or jog, skip for 3 minutes (can be performed stationary or moving)
2) Hip Circles (10 external rotations circles/leg)
3) Inchworms (10 reps)
4) Large arm circles (10 forward/10 backwards)
5) Standing spinal twists (20 twists)

Lower Body Exercises (Select One Each)

CATEGORY A	CATEGORY B
Squats	Floor Bridges
Plie Squats	Hamstring Bridges
Lunges	Donkey Kicks
Side Lunges	Fire Hydrants

Upper Body Exercises (Select One Each)

CATEGORY C	CATEGORY D
Pushups	Bicep Curl
Chest Fly	Hammer Curl
Shoulder Press	Tricep Extensions
Shoulder Fly	Tricep Dips
Back Fly	
Single-Arm Row	

Core/Abdominal Exercises (Choose Two)

CATEGORY E
Hover Plank
Crunch
Reverse Crunch
Bicycles
Side Plank
Quadruped
Super Man

Cardiovascular Exercises (Select Three)

CATEGORY F
Jumping Jacks
Squat Thrusts
Squat Jumps
High Knees
Mountain Climbers

HIIT Cardio

Perform one of these high intensity intervals (HIIT) on designated days. All HIIT circuits can be modified for different equipment. You can walk, jog, bike, stair climb, jump rope, use the elliptical or select any exercise from Category F to perform for your high intensity intervals. As you progress, feel free to increase the duration of the high intensity interval and/or decrease the duration of the moderate intensity interval.

You can use the Calendar Diet Intensity Scale to measure your exercise intensity. While exercising simply rate how hard you feel like you are working. This feeling should reflect how heavy and strenuous the exercise feels to you, combining all sensations and feelings of physical stress, effort, and fatigue. While you're exercising take a look at the rating scale below.

The scale ranges from 1 to 10, with 1 being "not working hard at all" to 10 meaning "working my hardest. Then choose the number that best describes your level of exertion. This will give you a good idea of the intensity level of your activity, which you can use to speed up or slow down your movements to reach your desired range.

THE CALENDAR DIET INTENSITY SCALE

1 = Not Working Hard At All
2
3
4
5 = Working Pretty Hard (Can still carry on a conversation)
6
7
8
9
10 = Working My Hardest (Maximal effort)

Listed on the next page are four HIIT interval training recommendations, but you can make up your own.

HIIT Interval A

	LEVEL 1	LEVEL 2	
Warm Up	5 min Warm up (fast walk, jog, bicycle, elliptical)	5 min Warm up (fast walk, jog, bicycle, elliptical)	
High Intensity Interval (RPE: 9-10)	30 seconds	30 seconds	
Moderate Intensity Interval (RPE: 5-6)	30 seconds	30 seconds	
# of Rounds	10	12	
Warm Down	As needed	As needed	
Total Time	20 minutes	12 - 18 minutes	

HIIT Interval B

	LEVEL 1	LEVEL 2	
Warm Up	5 min Warm up (fast walk, jog, bicycle, elliptical)	5 min Warm up (fast walk, jog, bicycle, elliptical)	
High Intensity Interval (RPE: 9-10)	20 seconds	30 seconds	
Moderate Intensity Interval (RPE: 5-6)	40 seconds	20 - 30 seconds	
# of Rounds	8	8	
Rest	2 minutes	2 minutes	
High Intensity Interval (RPE: 9-10)	20 seconds	30 seconds	
Moderate Intensity Interval (RPE: 5-6)	40 seconds	30 - 60 seconds	
# of Rounds	8	8	
Warm Down	As needed	As needed	
Total Time	18 minutes	13 - 18 minutes	

HIIT Interval C

	LEVEL 1	LEVEL 2	
Warm Up	5 min Warm up (fast walk, jog, bicycle, elliptical)	5 min Warm up (fast walk, jog, bicycle, elliptical)	
High Intensity Interval (RPE: 9-10)	1 minute	1 minute	
Moderate Intensity Interval (RPE: 5-6)	1 minute	1 minute	
# of Rounds	8 - 10	10 - 12	
Warm Down	As needed	As needed	
Total Time	16 - 20 minutes	18 - 20 minutes	

HIIT Interval D – Treadmill Hill Climb (Brisk Walk or Jog)

	LEVEL 1	LEVEL 2	
Warm Up	5 min Warm up (fast walk, jog)	5 min Warm up (fast walk, jog, bicycle, elliptical)	
High Intensity Interval (RPE: 9-10)	1 min/8 - 10% incline	1 min/10 - 12% incline	
Moderate Intensity Interval (RPE: 5-6)	1 min/2 - 3% incline	1 min/4 - 5% incline	
# of Rounds	10	10 - 12	
Warm Down	As needed	As needed	
Total Time	20 minutes	20 - 24 minutes	

Pyramid Training:

If you'd like to boost your cardiovascular endurance, but don't quite feel quite ready for cardio HIIT training, Pyramid Training is a great alternative. Warm-up for 5 minutes at a low intensity (3/10 on the work scale). Then increase the intensity level by 1 on the work scale (incline/speed/cadence) every 1 to 3 minutes, until you reach your maximum intensity (10/10 on the work scale). Next, decrease your intensity by 1 every 1 to 3 minutes. If you have time, repeat this again. Your total time should be 15 to 45 minutes/pyramid depending on the time you spend at each level.

Active Recovery:

On Active Recovery days give your body a chance to bounce back but still keep you active. Choose an activity you can do continuously for 30 to 60 minutes at a moderate (4/10 - 6/10) intensity level such as light jogging, easy bike ride, brisk walking.

Exercise Descriptions

Warm-Up Exercises:

1) Hip Circles – Standing on your right leg, bend your left leg to a 90 degree angle and rotate your knee in a counter-clockwise circle. Repeat for 10 reps.
Switch and stand on your left leg, rotating your right knee clockwise.

2) Inchworms – Begin in push-up position. Slowly walk your legs to your hands. Then slowly walk your hands forward until you are back in push-up position. Repeat for 10 reps.

3) Large Arm Circles – Stand with your feet shoulder width apart, with straight arms and your palms facing towards the ground. Rotate your arms
forward in large circles. Then reverse direction.

4) Standing Spinal Twists – Stand with your feet shoulder width apart. Extend your straight arms to shoulder level and rotate your body at the waist towards the right. Then pass through center to the left. Repeat.

Lower Body Exercises

Squat -

Stand with your feet slightly wider than shoulder-width apart, toes pointing forward. Lower your body as far as you can by pushing your hips back and bending your knees as if you were sitting on a chair. Drop to parallel or slightly below parallel, keeping your head up and back flat. Make sure that your knees stay behind the toes. Return to standing position.

(Advanced Option: Hold dumbbells in each hand with your arms extended on the outside of each leg. Your palms should face each other while performing the squat).

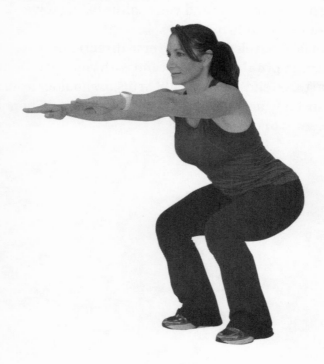

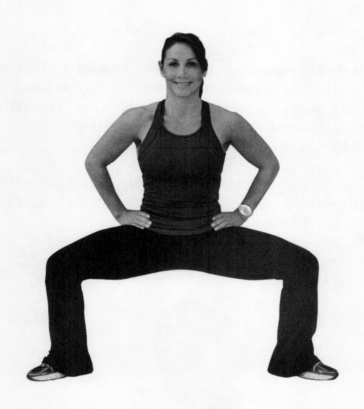

Plie Squat –

Stand with your feet wider than shoulder-width apart and toes pointed out to the side. Bend your knees and lower into a squat, keeping your knees in line with your toes. Return to starting position & repeat.

(Advanced Option: Hold dumbbells in each hand with your arms extended in between your legs. Your palms should face each other while performing the squat).

Lunge –

Begin in standing position. Step forward with your right leg and slowly bend both knees getting as close to the floor as possible (your front knee shouldn't go past your toe and both knees should bend to 90 degrees). Push yourself back up to the starting position and switch sides.

(Advanced Option: Hold dumbbells in each hand with arms extended on the outside of each leg. Your palms should face each other while performing the lunge).

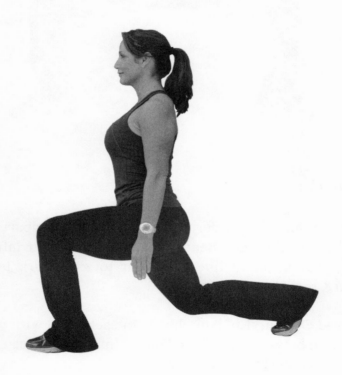

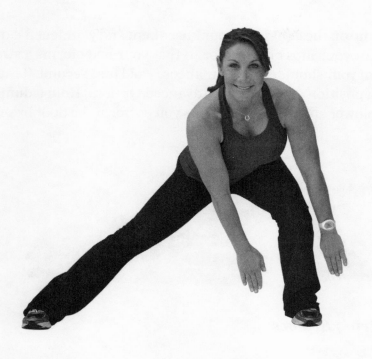

Side Lunge –

Stand with your feet shoulder-width apart. Take a big step with your left foot and push your hips back as you lower your body by bending your left knee as far as you can. Return to standing position and repeat on the same side until time is completed. Switch sides and repeat.

(Advanced Option: Hold dumbbells in each hand with arms extended on the outside of each leg. Your palms should face each other while performing the lunge. As you lunge to one side allow your arms to travel over to the side of the bent leg, placing your hands by that foot).

Floor Bridges –

Lie face up on the floor with your knees bent and your feet flat on the floor. Lift your hips off the floor so that your body forms a straight line from your shoulders to your knees. Hold for 1 second. Return to starting position and repeat. (Advanced Option: Hold a dumbbell on your lower abdomen/hip area as you perform the floor bridge).

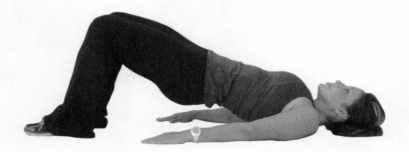

Hamstring Bridges –

Lie face up on the floor, bend your legs to a 90-degree angle and place your heels on a chair. Contract your glutes and lift your hips off the floor as high as possible, forming a straight line from your shoulders to your knees. Return to starting position and repeat. (Advanced option: Extend one leg up in the air and perform a single leg hamstring bridge. Switch sides and repeat).

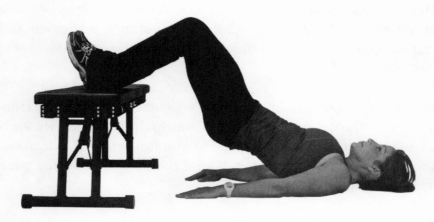

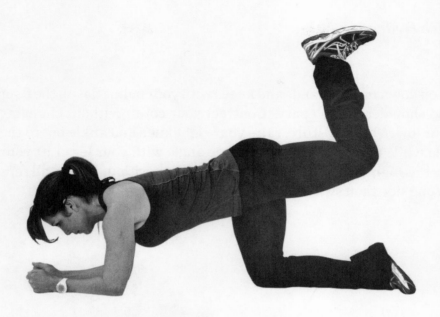

Donkey Kicks –

Kneel on a mat or soft surface on your hands and knees. Your palms should be flat on the floor and shoulder-width apart. Contract your core. Without changing your lower-back posture, raise your right knee and ankle towards the ceiling while maintaining a 90-degree angle with that leg. Return to starting position. Repeat all reps on one side then switch sides and repeat.

Fire Hydrants –

Drop down to your hands and knees with your palms flat on the floor and shoulder-width apart. Contract your core. Without changing your lower-back posture, raise your right knee and ankle out to the side while maintaining a 90- degree angle with your leg. Lift your knee as high as possible. Return to starting position. Repeat all reps on one side then switch sides & repeat.

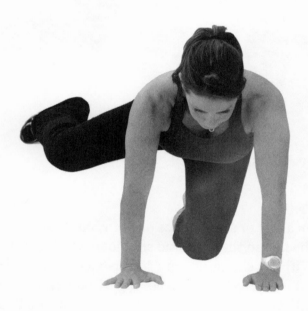

Upper Body Exercises:

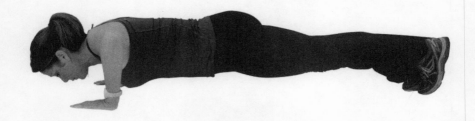

Pushups –

Get down on all fours and place your hands slightly wider than shoulder-width apart and in line with your shoulders. Straighten your legs and rise on to the balls of your feet so that your weight is supported by only your hands and feet. Bend your elbows and lower your body until your chest nearly touches the floor. Pause and return to starting position.

(Beginner Option: Perform the push-up on your knees with your heels pointed toward the ceiling.

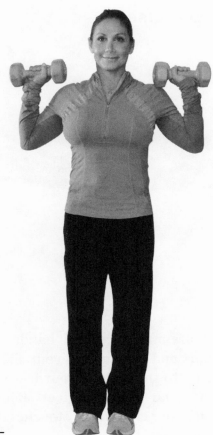

Shoulder Press –

Stand with your feet shoulder-width apart with a dumbbell in each hand. Begin with the arms bent so that the dumbbells rest just above your shoulders, palms facing forward. Press the dumbbells up until that are straight overhead. Return to starting position and repeat.

Chest Fly –

Lie face up on a bench or the floor with your knees bent and your feet flat on the floor or the bench. Holding a dumbbell in each hand, extend your arms toward the ceiling, palms facing each other and elbows slightly bent. Bring the dumb bells away from each other toward the ground as if you were giving someone a big hug. Return to starting position and repeat.

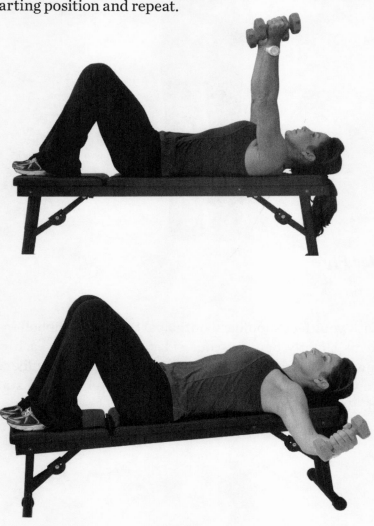

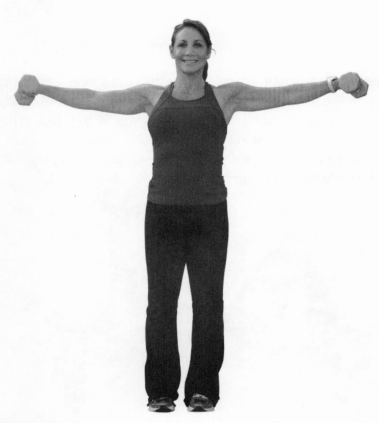

Shoulder Fly -

Stand with your feet shoulder-width apart with a dumbbell in each hand, arms slightly bent by your sides, palms facing each other. Keeping a slight bend in your arms, raise your arms to shoulder level, palms towards the floor. Pause and slowly lower arms to starting position. Repeat.

Back Fly –

Stand with your feet shoulder-width apart with a dumbbell in each hand. Contract your abdominals. Slightly bend your knees and bend forward at the waist keeping a flat back. Extend your arms towards the floor, palms facing each other. With slightly bent arms, raise each arm out to the side as if you were trying to fly. Pause and slowly and lower arms to starting position.Repeat.

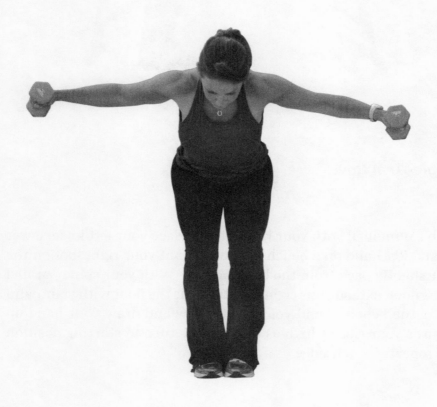

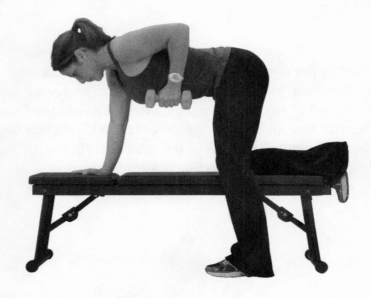

Single-Arm Row –

Grab a dumbbell with your right hand. Place your left knee, lower leg and left hand on a bench or chair. Plant your right foot on the floor slightly back from the bench/chair. With your spine parallel to the floor, extend your right arm towards the floor with your palm facing the bench. Bend your right elbow and draw your hand up towards your ribs as high as possible. Return to starting position and repeat. Switch sides.

Bicep Curl -

Stand with your feet shoulder-width apart, knees slightly bent, abdominals held tight. Hold a dumbbell or a band in each hand, arms extended by your sides, palms facing forward. Bend your arms at the elbows toward your shoulders. Keeping your elbows stationary, straighten to starting position and repeat.

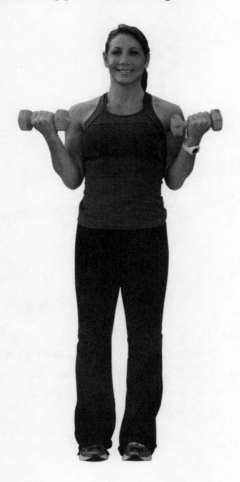

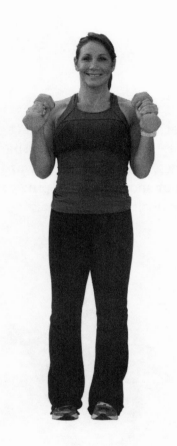

Hammer Curl -

Stand with your feet shoulder-width apart, knees slightly bent, abdominals held tight. Hold a dumbbell or a band in each hand, arms extended, palms facing each other. Bend your arms at the elbows toward your shoulders. Keeping the elbows stationary, straighten to starting position and repeat.

Tricep Extensions –

Lie face-up on the floor or a bench with your knees bent and your feet flat on the floor. Hold two dumbbells at arms' length over your upper chest, palms face each other. Bend the elbows lowering the dumbbells to the side of your head keeping the upper arm stationary. Extend the arms back to starting position and repeat.

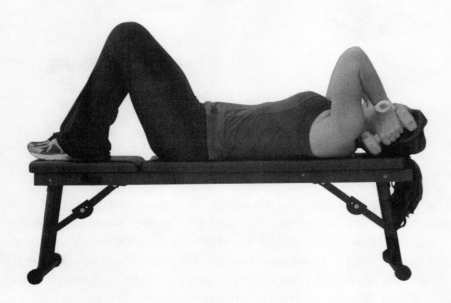

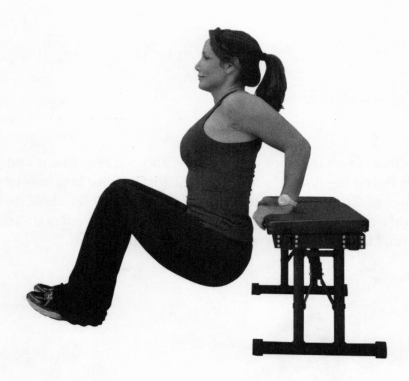

Tricep Dips -

Sit on the edge of a chair with your hands underneath your buttocks with your fingers facing forward and your palms down. Walk your feet out a couple of steps until your bottom is off the chair and your arms are straight. Lower your bodies just in front of the chair until your elbows are bent to 90 degrees. Then press through your palms, straighten your arms and return to starting position. Repeat.

Core Exercises:

Hover Plank –

Lie on your stomach on an exercise mat or soft surface. Prop your body up on your forearms and the balls of your feet. Your body should form a straight line from your shoulders to your ankles. Tighten your core by contracting your abdominals. Hold this position for the desired time.

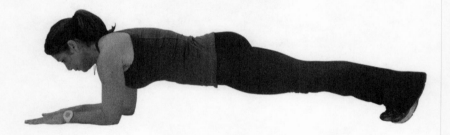

Crunch -

Lie face-up on the floor with your knees bent and your feet flat on the floor. Place your hands behind your head with your elbows pointing out to the sides. Contract your abdominals and lift your shoulders off the floor. Hold for 1 second and return to starting position. Repeat.

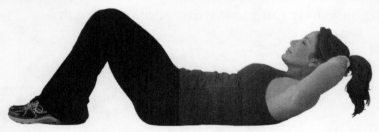

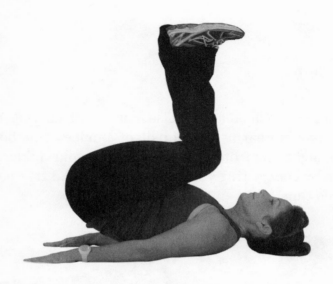

Reverse Crunch –

Lie face-up on the floor with your feet in the air and legs bent at a
90 degree angle. Place your hands, palms down on the floor by your
hips. Contract your abs and lift your hips off the floor as high as
possible keeping your legs bent at the same angle through the entire
movement, pause and return to starting position. Repeat.

Bicycles –

Lie face-up on the floor with your hands behind the head and your legs in a chair position. Lift your shoulders off the floor and twist your upper body to the left as you pull your left knee in towards the right elbow and simultaneously extend the right leg. Quickly return to starting position and repeat on the other side.

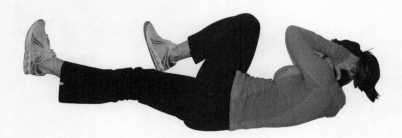

Side Plank –

Lie on your left side with your knees straight. Prop your upper body up on your left elbow and forearm. Raise your hips so that you are balancing on the side of the left foot and your forearm. Hold for the designated period of time. Switch sides and repeat.

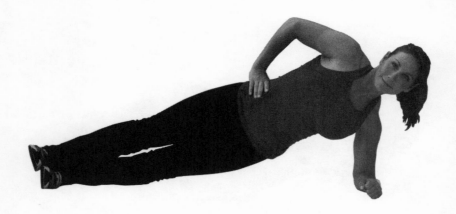

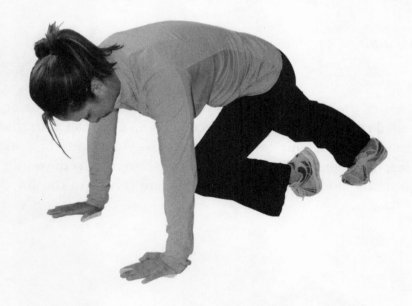

Quadruped –

Kneel on a mat or soft surface on your hands & knees. Contract your abdominals and without changing your lower back posture, simultaneously extend your right arm and left leg forming a straight line from your left foot to your right arm. Slowly return to starting position and switch sides.

Superman –

Lie face-down on the floor with your legs straight and your arms extended over your head palms faced down. Contract your glutes and the muscles of your lower back, and raise your head, chest, arms and legs off the floor. Your hips should be the only part of your body touching the floor. Hold for 3 seconds and return to the starting position.

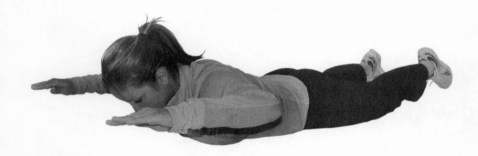

Cardiovascular Exercises:

Jumping Jacks –

Stand with your feet together and your hands by your sides. Simultaneously extend your arms above your head as you jump your legs out wide. Quickly return to starting position and repeat.

Squat Jumps –

From standing position, press your hips and bend your knees as low as possible while swinging your arms back in preparation to jump into the air. From this position, quickly jump as high as you can and extend your arms up over your head. Land into a squat position and repeat.

High Knees –

From standing position, hop onto your right leg and bend your left knee to 90 degrees driving it as high as possible towards your chest. Quickly hop onto your left leg and repeat.

Squat Thrusts –

Stand with your feet shoulder-width apart and your arms at your sides. Push your hips back, bend your knees into a squat position and lower your body placing your hands on the floor in front of you. Hop your legs backwards so that you are in push-up position; quickly bring your legs back into a squat position and return to standing position with a hop.

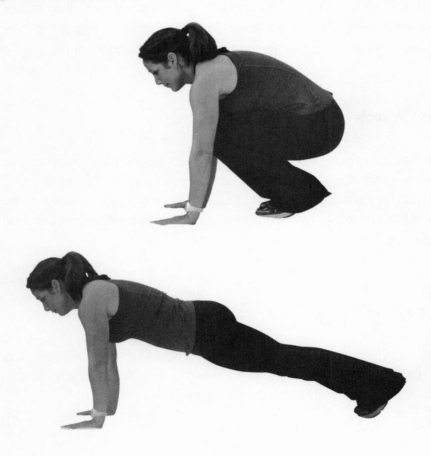

Mountain Climbers –

Place your hands on the floor slightly wider than shoulder-width apart and in line with your shoulders. Support your weight only on the balls of your feet and your hands. Your body should be in a straight line from your shoulders to your ankles. Bend your left leg bringing it towards your chest. Quickly bring it back to starting position while bringing your right leg to your chest. Repeat briskly.

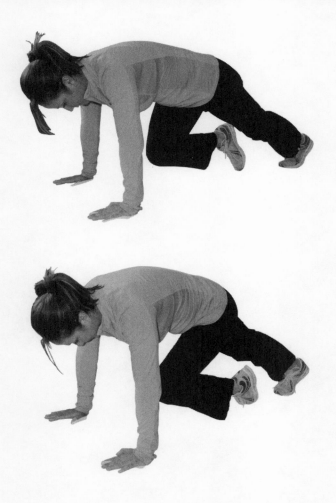

four
Appendices

Appendix A: Homework Section

January (or which ever month you start the diet)

WHAT DOES LOSING WEIGHT MEAN TO YOU?
Be specific and really think about this question. You can add to this list throughout the year.

1. _____

_____

2. _____

_____

3. _____

_____

4. _____

_____

5. _____

_____

6. _____

_____

March Homework: (or 2 months after you start the diet)

List 5 things that you've accomplished over the past 2 months. This doesn't only have to be weight loss related (ie: got to the gym three times this week, cooked three new vegetables, made healthier compromises eating out – be specific)

1. _____

2. _____

3. _____

4. _____

5. _____

Now list 3 things that you want to accomplish over the next month and check off when completed. (Repeat this exercise every 1-2 months)

Month:

☐ _____

_____

_____

☐ _____

_____

_____

☐ _____

_____

Month:

☐ _____

_____

_____

☐ _____

_____

_____

☐ _____

_____

_____

Month:

☐ _____

_____

_____

☐ _____

_____

_____

☐ _____

_____

_____

Month:

☐ _____

_____

_____

☐ _____

_____

_____

☐ _____

_____

_____

Month:

☐ _____

_____

_____

☐ _____

_____

_____

☐ _____

_____

_____

Month:

☐ _____

_____

_____

☐ _____

_____

_____

☐ _____

_____

_____

Month:

☐ _____

_____

_____

☐ _____

_____

_____

☐ _____

_____

_____

Appendix B:
Tips For Dining Out

Since we eat roughly 30% of our meals away from home, no diet book would be truly complete without advice on how to eat out while dieting. Here are some tips to keep in mind when eating out as well as specific suggestions for different types of restaurants.

General Tips:

• Consider ordering one or two appetizers instead of an entrée. Or, order an appetizer and a salad. You can also order items a la carte to keep portions and calories under control.
• Start smart. Research shows that having a low calorie soup or salad before meals can help you eat significantly fewer calories. Just stay away from cream-based soups and gobs of calorie-filled salad dressing and high fat salad toppings like cheese, nuts, croutons or bacon.
• If you're craving a main dish that's not the healthiest choice, start with a salad (dressing on the side) or light appetizer. Then share the entrée you're craving with your friend or
significant other.
• If the portion size you are served is too big, put half in a to go box before you get started. That way you won't inadvertently eat more than you planned to.
• Ask A LOT of questions if you don't know how a dish is prepared. When in doubt, always ask for sauce on the side so you can decide how much you want to eat.

- Swap sides. If a dish comes with potatoes or rice, ask for vegetables instead – just make sure they aren't drowning in oil.
- Skip the bread. Don't be shy about asking the waiter not to bring it. If your dining partner balks, tell him or her to keep it on their side of the table out of your reach.
- Make trade-offs whenever you can. If you're having wine, skip the bread. If you want dessert, skip the second glass of wine. Every good decision counts!

Dining Out: Specific Suggestions

Fast Food:

- Always go for grilled. Don't assume that breaded chicken or fish are lower in calories than beef.
- Consider eating burgers and sandwiches topless to save up to 100 calories
- Watch the sauces and toppings – they can add hundreds of calories.
- Watch out for high calorie salads – dressings, breaded chicken and extra toppings (think non-vegetables) can easily add up to more calories than a burger.
- Share sides. If you have to have fries, get a small and split them.
- Watch the breakfast breads – croissants and biscuits are loaded with calories. Stick with an English muffin or flat bread.
- Skip the soda and sweetened tea.

Mexican:

- Watch the cheese and sour cream. These often come standard on Mexican food so ask for light cheese if you can. If you can't, skip it entirely.
Ditto for the sour cream or go for a little guacamole instead.

- Order a burrito bowl instead of a burrito. The tortilla alone packs up to 300 calories. Skip the rice and stick with beans, guacamole and chicken or shrimp, and order salsa as your dressing.
- Hard taco shells are actually lower in calories than soft tacos.
- If you can avoid it, don't get started eating chips. It's too hard to limit yourself to one serving.
- Choose whole beans instead of refried beans
- Choose red or green sauces instead of cream or cheese sauces.

Italian:

- Start with minestrone soup or salad and order an appetizer portion of pasta. This leaves room for a glass of wine, a shared dessert, or a small piece of bread.
- Watch the cheese and sauce. Go for marinara, not alfredo, carbonara, or pesto.
- Avoid breaded dishes like parmigiana or fried appetizers like calamari.
- If a dish comes with a side of pasta, ask for steamed or lightly sautéed vegetables instead.

Chinese:

- Always go for dishes that are steamed not fried, crispy, or breaded.
- Ask for brown rice if available. If not, limit your portion of rice to the size of a baseball.
- Ask for dry wok if possible (minimal oil is used)
- Start with soup.
- Watch out for dishes with nuts as they can add hundreds of extra calories.

Deli/Sandwiches:

• Avoid mayonnaise-based sandwiches as they're loaded with hidden calories (i.e. tuna salad, chicken salad, egg salad).
• Eat half of the bread whenever possible – especially for sandwiches that are served on a huge deli roll.
• Skip the cheese and mayo and go for avocado and/or Dijon mustard instead.
• Don't automatically order chips. One of my patients surprised herself when she realized that she didn't really need them to feel satisfied.

Pizza:

• Pack on the vegetable toppings and skip high fat meats like sausage and pepperoni.
• Ask for thin crust (whole wheat if available) and light cheese – it could save you hundreds of calories.
• Start with a big salad (dressing on the side) to fill up faster.

Sushi:

• Ask for light rice (they use less to wrap the roll) and save hundreds of calories effortlessly.
• Start with miso soup and/or edamame.
• Cut back on rolls with fried filling (spider roll) and mayonnaise (spicy tuna roll).
• Sashimi is always a great (although slightly more expensive).

Steak House:

• Filet mignon and sirloin are the leanest.
• Limit the toppings on your potato to a little butter (think

no more than a pat) or a soup spoon full of sour cream for flavor.

- Go for steamed instead of creamed vegetables.
- Consider starting with soup or salad (dressing on the side) and splitting a steak – even half of an 8-ounce steak is plenty for most people.

Brunch Buffet:

- Survey the buffet before you start filling your plate. This will allow you to decide which healthy foods you are going to fill up on and which small splurges to indulge in.
- Omelet bars are terrific – just ask for light oil (or non-stick spray if they have it) and loads of vegetables. You can even have a tablespoon of shredded cheese.
- Watch out for healthy-sounding yogurt with granola. More often that not, this is full-fat yogurt loaded with sugar and high-fat granola.
- Watch the pastries, muffins, sweet breads. Splurge by having one if you must but don't load your plate with several telling yourself that you will just have a bite of each!

Salad Bars:

- Limit the higher calorie toppings like nuts, cheese, seeds, dried fruit and croutons as these can easily add up to 500 extra calories. Choose your favorite and allow yourself one soupspoon full. You can use these same guidelines when ordering a salad at a restaurant.
- Always get the dressing on the side unless you are drizzling olive oil (limit this to 1 tablespoon) and vinegar on the salad. A quarter-cup of dressing (even balsamic vinaigrette) can easily pack 180 to 300 calories.
- Skip the mayonnaise-filled salads like tuna salad, chicken salad, pasta salad, and egg salad.

Appendix C:
Tips For Boosting Weight Loss Or Busting Through Plateaus

If you're feeling especially motivated to lose weight or have reached a plateau, try these tips to help you lose weight more quickly or get the number on the scale moving in the right direction again.

• **Double your non-starchy vegetable intake** and cut bread,grains, and starchy vegetables in half. This will help you automatically cut calories while boosting your nutritional intake. To make this easy, choose from the low carb seasonal options.

• **Limit the amount you eat out.** I know it's not easy, but you have much more control over what you eat when you eat at home. If you have to eat out, keep it simple. The 'cleaner' the dish (ie. the fewer the sauces, toppings, etc.) the fewer the hidden calories.

• **Track everything.** If you stopped keeping a journal, or never started, start tracking everything you eat and how much you exercise. You might be surprised to find that you have more calorie amnesia than you realized.

• **Cut liquid calories.** It is amazing how quickly the calories in coffee drinks, bottled teas and waters, and alcohol add up. If you really want to see the number on the scale move, cut these for a few weeks and fill up on food instead.

• **Split workouts and up the intensity.** Research shows that when you exercise more intensely, your body burns more calories for up to 14 hours afterwards. If you can swing it, consider working out twice a day, and up the intensity when you can.

Appendix D:
Calendar Kitchen Essentials

This list can help you get your kitchen "Calendar friendly". Stock your fridge and pantry with these basic ingredients (mostly non-perishable) to make cooking calendar meals easy. The only ingredients you'll need to fill in with are the freshest ones like seasonal produce and proteins like meat, chicken or fish.

Refrigerator:

o   Eggs
o   Non-fat milk
o   Non-fat plain Greek yogurt
o   Non-fat ricotta cheese
o   1% cottage cheese
o   Reduced-fat sour cream
o   Shredded reduced-fat cheddar cheese
o   Shredded reduced-fat mozzarella cheese
o   Unsalted butter
o   Blue cheese crumbles
o   Feta cheese crumbles
o   Grated Parmesan cheese
o   Marinara sauce
o   Low-sodium soy sauce
o   Worcestershire sauce
o   Ketchup
o   Dijon mustard

- o Barbeque sauce
- o Mango chutney
- o Salsa (regular and tomatillo)
- o Pesto
- o Peanut butter (smooth and chunky)
- o Almond butter
- o All fruit orange marmalade
- o Lemons
- o Limes
- o Orange juice
- o Pomegranate juice
- o Capers
- o Salad dressing (balsamic vinaigrette, honey mustard, Italian,Asian vinaigrette)

Pantry:

- o Brown rice
- o Whole-wheat penne
- o Whole-wheat spaghetti
- o Whole-wheat rotini
- o Whole-wheat couscous
- o Elbow macaroni
- o Polenta
- o Quinoa
- o Quick cooking and rolled oats
- o Low-sodium chicken or vegetable broth
- o Agave nectar
- o Honey
- o Sugar
- o Maple syrup
- o Brown sugar
- o Rice wine vinegar
- o Balsamic vinegar
- o Non-stick cooking spray

- Canola, olive, & sesame oil
- Canned diced green chili peppers
- Canned diced tomatoes
- Tomato paste
- Canned no-salt-added beans (chickpeas, cannellini, pinto, black)
- Canned pumpkin
- Canned tuna in water
- Roast peppers in jar
- Golden raisins
- Dried apricots
- Sliced almonds
- Chopped walnuts
- Sunflower seeds
- White wine
- Sherry
- Panko
- Bread crumbs
- Semisweet chocolate chips
- Whole-wheat pita chips

Spice Rack:

- Cumin
- Garlic powder
- Chili powder
- Curry powder
- Dried oregano
- Dried basil
- Dried coriander
- Cinnamon
- Ground nutmeg
- Red pepper flakes
- Wasabi or wasabi paste
- Kosher salt
- Pepper

Bread drawer:

o   Whole-wheat hamburger buns
o   Whole-wheat bread
o   Corn tortillas
o   Whole wheat tortillas
o   Whole-wheat deli flats
o   Whole-wheat bagel flats
o   Whole-wheat pita bread
o   Whole-wheat pizza crust

Freezer:

o   Whole grain waffles
o   Frozen peas
o   Frozen edamame
o   Frozen corn
o   Frozen peaches
o   Frozen raspberries

Appendix E:
Supplementing Your Diet

The Calendar Diet is packed with nutrients, so you're probably getting most, if not all, of what you need from your diet. However, I do recommend supplements to most of my patients who are restricting calories and who want to achieve optimal health. When choosing supplements, it's important to go with a reputable company that has rigorous quality control standards in place to ensure that you're getting exactly what it says on the label. If possible, look for products carrying the USP (United States Pharmacopoeia) or NSF third party verification seal.

Here is a list of the supplements that I recommend. Make sure to discuss your personal supplement requirements with your physician.

Basic Multivitamin/Mineral Supplement –

When we cut calories, we often reduce nutrient intake. I recommend a basic multivitamin supplement to all of my patients to ensure that they are getting everything that they need on a daily basis. I don't recommend taking mega doses of any individual vitamin or mineral.

Fish Oil (Omega 3 Fatty Acids) –

I've been a huge fan of omega 3 fatty acids for years. The range of potential benefit of omega 3 fatty acids is extensive and includes heart health, brain health, decreased risk of depression, improved immunity, and more. Omega 3 fatty acids are essential fatty acids, meaning your body cannot produce them. If you don't eat fatty fish like salmon at least twice a week, I recommend taking 1,000 mg of fish oil daily for optimal health. If you have high triglycerides, rheumatoid arthritis, or other inflammatory conditions, talk to your doctor about potentially taking higher doses.

Calcium/Vitamin D –

These are critical for bone health if you are trying to lose weight and don't consume three servings of dairy every day. For most of my patients I recommend 1,000 IU of vitamin D3 and either 500mg of calcium if you regularly eat dairy products and drink milk, or 1,000 mg calcium if you don't.

If you take antacids or acid blocking medication regularly, you might consider taking calcium citrate instead of calcium carbonate for improved absorption. If you do eat plenty of dairy but don't get enough Vitamin D (risk factors for vitamin D deficiency include living in northern latitudes, African American ethnicity, obesity and age greater than 65), I definitely recommend a vitamin D supplement. Talk with your doctor to have your Vitamin D levels checked.

Probiotics –

I'm a big believer in the benefits of probiotics for optimal health. If you don't eat probiotic-fortified foods such as yogurt or kefir, you might consider taking a daily supplement, particularly if you have digestive difficulties or get frequent colds. Look for a supplement with multiple strains of probiotics as different strains have different functions.

B Complex –

If you don't feel like you need a multivitamin, I recommend taking a B complex supplement to ensure that you get all the energy-boosting B vitamins you need on a daily basis. In addition, if you're over the age of 65, you may not absorb Vitamin B 12 as effectively so a B complex supplement can ensure adequate B12 intake. If you are a woman of child-bearing age, getting adequate amounts of folic acid (at least 400 mcg a day) is critical for preventing neural tube defects should you get pregnant.

Plant Sterols –

These are naturally occurring plant compounds that help lower cholesterol. If you have high cholesterol and it is not responding adequately to The Calendar Diet and weight loss, you might want to consider taking a plant sterol supplement. The FDA recommends 2 grams per day for cholesterol reductions. I prefer a supplement instead of fortified foods in order to limit additional calories (unless the fortified food is replacing a food that's already in your diet and isn't) an additional source of calories.

Unfortunately, a safe and effective weight loss supplement does not exist. There has been some researching suggesting that a combination of caffeine and green tea extract may help with weight loss, but due to the variability in product formulations and doses, it is very difficult to recommend a specific product. Most products claiming to boost metabolism or fat burning have not been proven clinically therefore I do not recommend them.

Appendix F:
Tips for Tackling Frozen Meals

Frozen meals can be a smart way to control calories and portion size when you don't have time to cook. Here's what to look for:

1. Look for meals that are around 250 – 400 calories (depending on meal and your size).
2. Make sure they contain at least 3 to 5 grams of fiber.
3. Aim for 10 grams of protein or more.
4. Aim for less than 4 grams of saturated fat.
5. Try to limit sodium to less than 600 mg.
6. Look for meals that have vegetables listed in the top half of
    the ingredient list to make sure that not all of the carbohydrates in the meal come from grains.
7. Try to choose products that use whole grains like brownrice or whole wheat pasta when they are available.

About the authors

Melina B. Jampolis, M.D.

Dr. Melina is one of only several hundred board certified physician nutrition specialists in the United States. A graduate of Tufts University and Tufts University School of medicine, she completed her internal medicine residency at Santa Clara Valley Medical Center, a Stanford University teaching hospital. She is a member of the American Society for Nutrition and the Obesity Society.

She was the host of Fit Tv's Diet Doctor (Discovery Communications) and has served as the diet and fitness expert for CNN.com since 2008. Her first book, The No Time to Lose Diet (Nelson Books) was released in 2007. She is a frequent guest on national television programs including Live with Regis and Kelly, Dr. Oz, Fox Business Network and CNN and is regularly interviewed for diet and nutrition related publications across the country.

She lives and works in Los Angeles with her husband, 2 year old son Max, and dogs Rusty and Jezebel. She has a passion for wine and is currently a spinning/yoga fanatic.

Karen Ansel, M.S., R.D., C.D.N.

is a nutrition consultant, journalist and author specializing in nutrition, health and wellness. She is a regular contributor to national women's, health and cooking magazines and is the co-author of Healthy in a Hurry (Weldon Owen, January 2012) and the 2011 IACP finalist The Baby & Toddler Cookbook: Fresh, Homemade Foods for a Healthy Start (Weldon Owen, 2010).

She is a spokesperson for the Academy of Nutrition and Dietetics and a contributing editor for Woman's Day Magazine. Karen is a graduate of Duke University and she received her Masters of Science in clinical nutrition from New York University.

Karen lives in Long Island, New York with her husband and two daughters ages 12 and 17. When she's not busy writing about nutrition, she enjoys cooking, running and playing with her dog, Cosmo.

Ami Jampolis, M.S, CSCS

is the owner of Focus Fitness and a certified personal trainer through the National Association of Sports Medicine as well as a Certified Strength & Conditioning Specialist. She has over 17 years experience in the health & fitness industry. Ami holds a Bachelor's Degree in Kinesiology and a Master's Degree in Exercise Physiology from Arizona State University. She spent several years working in physical therapy learning injury prevention & rehabilitation which she incorporates into her personal training. She lives in Northern California with her adorable son, Colten James.